THE HANDBOOK OF SEXUAL HEALTH IN PRIMARY CARE

Editors   Toni Belfield
Yvonne Carter
Philippa Matthews
Catti Moss
Anne Weyman

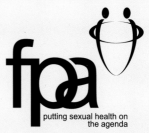

fpa

putting sexual health on
the agenda

First edition published 1998 by The Royal College of General Practitioners.

Published by **fpa**
2–12 Pentonville Road
London N1 9FP

Tel: 0845 122 8600
Fax: 0845 123 2349
www.fpa.org.uk

The Family Planning Association is a registered charity, number 250187 and a limited liability company registered in England, number 887632.

ISBN: 899194 82 7

Disclaimer
The information in this book is based on the evidence and medical opinion at the time of publication. Care has been taken to ensure that the information given in this text is accurate and up to date. Medical knowledge and practice is constantly changing, as new information becomes available, as such changes in treatment procedures and use of drugs or practice become necessary.

Printed by:
Jason Print and Design, Hertfordshire

Contents

Acknowledgements **5**

Table of abbreviations **7**

Foreword **9**
Sir Liam Donaldson

Introduction **11**
Toni Belfield, Yvonne Carter, Philippa Matthews, Catti Moss and *Anne Weyman*

1. Professional skill mix **19**
Catriona Sutherland, Shelley Mehigan and *Caroline Davey*

2. Risk assessment and sexual history-taking in primary care **35**
Philippa Matthews and *Rita Ireson*

3. Contraception **57**
Philip Hannaford

4. Pregnancy planning **121**
Tom Heyes

5. Abortion **137**
Kate Guthrie

6. Sexually transmissible infections: a primary care perspective **155**
Philippa Matthews and *Helen Macaulay*

7. The diagnosis of HIV in a primary care setting **187**
Philippa Matthews

8. Sexual dysfunction in primary care   **209**
Gill Wakley

9. Screening well people   **227**
Muir Gray and *Jennifer Hopwood*

10. Sexual health – learning from consumers   **245**
Toni Belfield

11. Evaluating sexual health service provision in general practice   **259**
Kaye Wellings

About the authors and editors   **273**

Index   **277**

Acknowledgements

We would like to thank the many people who have made this book possible. We are grateful to the Department of Health which generously provided funding for this second edition of the book, and to Sir Liam Donaldson for writing the foreword. Our heartfelt thanks also go to the authors who found time in their immensely busy professional lives to contribute to this book, and who have worked so hard to meet deadlines.

Much of the book, including the protocols, could not have been written without the support, and the willing sharing of expertise, by the staff of the following organisations:

- Lee Bank Group Practice (including primary care based sexual health outreach workers (SHOW)), South Birmingham PCT
- Sexual Health in Practice, Heart of Birmingham PCT
- West Midlands Deanery GP Unit.

We are also grateful to Blackwell Publishing for giving us permission to reproduce the graph in Chapter 7.

Our thanks also go to Jane Hobden, freelance editor, who prepared the text for publication, and to those **fpa** staff who have been involved in supporting this book's production in a myriad of ways.

Table of abbreviations

AIDS – acquired immune deficiency syndrome

ART – antiretroviral therapy

BMI – body mass index

BNF – British National Formulary

BV – bacterial vaginosis

CIN – cervical intraepithelial neoplasia

CLaSS – Chlamydia Screening Studies

COC – combined oral contraceptive

CMV – cytomegalovirus retinitis

D&C – dilatation and curettage

DMPA – depot medroxyprogesterone acetate

DVT – deep vein thrombosis

EC – emergency contraception

ED – everyday

EE – ethinyl estradiol

EHC – emergency hormonal contraception

ELISA – enzyme-linked immunosorbent assay

EPO – earliest predicted ovulation

GMS – General Medical Services

GP – general practitioner

GUM – genitourinary medicine

HAART – highly active anti-retroviral therapy

HCG – human chorionic gonadotrophin

HIV – human immunodeficiency virus

HPV – human papilloma virus

HSV – herpes simplex virus

IUD – intrauterine device

IUS – intrauterine system

IVDU– intravenous drug user

LAM – lactational amenorrhoea method

LMP – last menstrual period

MSU – mid-stream urine (sample)

NCSP – National Chlamydia Screening Programme

NSGI – non-specific genital infection

NSU – non-specific urethritis

NAAT – nucleic acid amplification test

NNRT – non nucleoside reverse transcriptase inhibitor

PCC – postcoital contraception

PCG – primary care group

PCO – primary care organisation

PCP – pneumocystis carinii pneumonia

PCR – polymerase chain reaction

PCT – primary care trust

PE – pulmonary embolism

PEP – post exposure prophylaxis

PGD – patient group directions

PHCT – primary healthcare team

PI – protease inhibitor

PID – pelvic inflammatory disease

PMS – personal medical services

PN – practice nurse

POP – progestogen-only pill

RCT – randomised controlled trials

RUQ – right upper quadrant

SDA – strand displacement amplification

SHOW – primary care based sexual health outreach worker

STI – sexually transmissible infection

TOC – tests of cure

TFI – tubal factor infertility

TV – Trichomonas vaginalis

UPSI – unprotected sexual intercourse

Foreword

I am delighted to see the second edition of this handbook for primary care practitioners, after the very successful first edition. Sexual health is an issue which has grown in significance over the past few years. With the publication of the Department of Health's *Sexual Health and HIV Strategy*, and the White Paper *Choosing Health*, both discussed further in the book's introduction, it has been identified as a key public health issue.

Sexual health is an important topic for the NHS, and increasingly, general practice is playing a larger role in the delivery of sexual health services. Using an evidence-based approach, this book provides clear, practical guidance which primary care practitioners will find easy to incorporate into their everyday practice. A broad range of topics is covered by a cross-section of authors respected in the field. It is especially pleasing to see issues addressed such as multidisciplinary working, risk assessment and management of problems, maintaining quality of service, and screening, along with topics such as HIV diagnosis, sexual problems and pregnancy planning.

I believe that this handbook will help primary care teams to deliver the best possible sexual health care to their patients, which in turn will make an important contribution to their local population's health and wellbeing.

Sir Liam Donaldson, Chief Medical Officer

Introduction

Toni Belfield, Yvonne Carter, Philippa Matthews, Catti Moss and Anne Weyman

Since the first edition of this handbook was published in 1998, sexual health has taken on much greater significance in the national agenda. In 1998, the Government launched its Teenage Pregnancy Strategy. Two years later, in 2000, the National Assembly for Wales published a Sexual Health Strategy for Wales. In 2001, the Department of Health in England published its National Strategy for Sexual Health and HIV, followed in 2002 by an action plan to implement the strategy. The Scottish Sexual Health Strategy was launched in early 2005 and the Northern Ireland strategy is awaited.

In 2003, the House of Commons Health Select Committee issued the report of its inquiry into sexual health. They identified a crisis in sexual health and called on the Government to improve services and raise awareness with the public. The Committee revisited its report in 2005 and again expressed concern about the situation. Rising levels of sexually transmissible infections (STIs) and the high rates of teenage pregnancy in the UK give rise to endless stories in the press, and the demand for services increases.

The Government's public health White Paper, *Choosing Health: Making healthy choices easier*, published in 2004, recognised these concerns and identified improving sexual health as a key public health issue. The White Paper promises:

- a new public awareness campaign targeted particularly at young men and women to highlight the risks of unprotected sex and to promote the use of condoms to protect against STIs or unplanned pregnancy

- an accelerated introduction of the national screening programme for chlamydia so that it covers the whole of England by 2007

- a review of contraceptive services in 2005 followed by investment to meet gaps in local services and, in particular, to ensure that the full range of contraceptive services is available, that good practice is spread and that services are modernised

- a goal, that by 2008, everyone referred to a genitourinary medicine (GUM) clinic should be able to have an appointment within 48 hours.

To fund these improvements, £300 million of new money has been allocated.

Supported by the Department of Health and after extensive consultation, in early 2005 The Medical Foundation for Aids and Sexual Health (MedFASH) published ten recommended standards for sexual health which are applicable to all settings including general practice. The standards provide markers of good practice to help improve quality and responsiveness to individual need.

Clearly these developments will have an impact on primary care and the services provided in general practice. However, the most significant change for practices that we have seen since the first edition of this book is the introduction of the General Medical Services (GMS) contractual arrangements within general practice across the UK which came into effect from 1 April 2004. The impact of the 2004 contract on sexual health services is as yet not fully known. However, it is becoming apparent that, in many areas, general practice is playing a bigger role in the delivery of sexual health services. The introduction of practice based commissioning will create a new environment for the increasing role of general practice in the future.

THE SEXUAL HEALTH STRATEGY

In England, the National Strategy for Sexual Health and HIV put forward a three-level system for sexual health services:

Level One services

- sexual history-taking and risk assessment
- contraceptive information and services
- STI testing for women
- assessment and referral of men with STI symptoms
- HIV testing and counselling
- cervical cytology screening and referral
- pregnancy testing and referral
- hepatitis B immunisation.

Level Two services

- intrauterine device insertion (IUD, IUS)
- contraceptive implant insertion
- testing and treating STIs
- partner notification
- STI testing for men.

Level Three services

- outreach for STI prevention
- outreach contraceptive services
- specialised infections management, including co-ordination of partner notification
- highly specialised contraception
- specialised HIV treatment and care.

The strategy envisaged that most practices would provide Level One services with the rest providing some or all of the elements of Level Two services. The strategy also suggests that services need to make patients feel that they can discuss problems with their sex lives, assess patients and refer on to specialist services where appropriate.

Level Three services and some of Levels One and Two services would be provided by family planning and GUM services. All service providers would be part of a network and the family planning and GUM providers would act as a source of support and advice to professionals in general practice.

GENERAL MEDICAL SERVICES CONTRACT

The 2004 GMS contract also has three different categories within it: *essential, additional* and *enhanced services*. However, these only overlap partially with the levels in the Sexual Health and HIV Strategy.

Essential services

The essential services, which all practices have to provide, involve managing patients and temporary residents who are:

- ill, or believe themselves to be ill, with conditions from which recovery is generally expected

- terminally ill
- suffering from chronic disease.

Practices also have to provide:

- advice in connection with the patient's health, including relevant health promotion advice, and
- referring the patient for other services.

The term 'management' includes:

- offering consultation and, where appropriate, physical examination for the purpose of identifying the need, if any, for treatment or further investigation
- making available such treatment or further investigation as is necessary and appropriate, including the referral of the patient for other services under the Act and liaison with other health care professionals involved in the patient's treatment and care.

Essential services from a sexual health point of view include a number of Level One services such as sexual history-taking, consultations about STIs, HIV, unwanted pregnancy, and referral to other services such as GUM or abortion services. They also include referral to psychosexual services.

Additional services

Additional services are those which the practice has a preferential right to provide, but the practice can decide to opt out of their provision as a means of managing their workload. There are seven additional services, including contraception and cervical cytology. In the case of contraception, the practice can also opt out for reasons of conscience. If a practice does opt out of providing any of the additional services, the funding allocated to them is retained by the primary care organisation (PCO) which becomes responsible for commissioning or for ensuring that patients receive the services from another provider.

If they are providing contraception as an additional service, the regulations require practices to offer the following services:

- giving advice about the full range of contraceptive methods
- where appropriate, the medical examination of patients seeking such advice
- treating such patients for contraceptive purposes and prescribing contraceptive substances and appliances (excluding the fitting and implanting of intrauterine devices and implants)

- giving advice about emergency contraception and where appropriate, supplying or prescribing emergency hormonal contraception. Where the contractor has a conscientious objection to emergency contraception, prompt referral must be given to another provider of primary medical services who does not have such conscientious objections

- providing advice and referral in cases of unplanned or unwanted pregnancy, including advice about the availability of free pregnancy testing in the practice area. Where the contractor has a conscientious objection to abortion, prompt referral must be given to another provider of primary medical services who does not have such conscientious objections

- giving initial advice about sexual health promotion and STIs

- referring as necessary for specialist sexual health services, including tests for STIs.

Although these regulations require the practice to give advice on all methods of contraception, they do not specify that the practice must provide intrauterine devices (IUDs and IUSs) and implants.

Improving quality of care: A key purpose of the contract is to improve the quality of primary care. A National Quality and Outcome Framework has been agreed which includes quality points for specific aspects of additional services. Practices can obtain additional payment if they achieve these. For contraception, there is one additional point available for practices with a written policy for emergency contraception. A further point is available for those with a written policy for pre-conceptual advice. This covers stopping a contraceptive method in anticipation of conceiving and areas such as smoking, alcohol, diet, prophylactic folic acid, rubella status, any genetically inherited condition, substance abuse and any existing medical condition. It has little to do with contraception. PCOs are responsible for performance managing the quality points claimed by a practice through annual monitoring of the practice.

Enhanced services

Enhanced services make up the third category of provision. There are three types of enhanced services: directed enhanced services, national enhanced services and local enhanced services. PCOs must commission all six of the directed enhanced services, none of which relates to sexual health. All other enhanced services are provided at the discretion of the PCO. The specifications and payment tariffs for national enhanced services are set nationally and those for local enhanced services are a matter for the PCO to agree locally. In the case of sexual health, there are currently two national enhanced services: IUD and More Specialised Sexual Health Services.

Implants are not included in national enhanced services, although the PCO is responsible for delivering the patient services guarantee which requires that patients continue to be offered at least the range of services that they have enjoyed under the previous GMS contract. Thus, if implants have been provided by practices previously, the PCO has to continue to commission this service but not necessarily from the same provider.

More specialised sexual health services include HIV and STI screening and treatment, the provision of condoms, pregnancy testing kits, prescriptions without charge for STI treatments, and partner notification programmes.

PCOs may choose to develop local enhanced services in a range of areas including expanding the provision of implants, young people's sexual health services, and training programmes to support all practices to provide Level One services as defined by the sexual health strategy.

PMS CONTRACTS

Personal medical services (PMS) contracts and budgets are not affected by the 2004 GMS contract and so PMS practices continue to provide services as specified in their PMS contracts. PMS practices have equivalent opportunities to opt out of additional services, to access the quality money, and to provide enhanced services. PMS practices may agree with the PCO a variation of the allocation of quality points to suit the profile of their patients. For example, a practice serving a largely student population can transfer quality points for coronary heart disease or diabetes to quality points for sexual health services such as chlamydia, STI and HIV testing.

Reviewing the GMS contract

As the 2004 contract differs significantly from previous arrangements, it is being kept under review during the first years of operation. It is to be hoped that these reviews will help to develop further the role of primary care in the provision of sexual health services, and that the range of enhanced sexual health services at both national and local levels will be extended. Furthermore, there is considerable scope for increasing the number of quality points for this area of work, especially with the completion of new standards of practice which are currently being developed.

TERMINOLOGY

The editors have endeavoured to use the most appropriate and up-to-date terminology throughout this book. For example the term 'sexually transmissible infection' is more specific than sexually transmitted infection or disease; 'abortion' has replaced 'termination of pregnancy' in professional guidance because it is the term that women prefer; and HIV is used in preference to the cumbersome HIV/AIDS for reasons explained in the chapter. We have not changed the term 'patient' to 'client' or 'service user' because 'patient' is so widely used and accepted by health professionals and the public alike. Chapter 11 is an exception because the context is different and necessitates a different approach.

The term 'primary care' is commonly used by GPs and practice nurses to denote general practice and related services provided by professionals such as health visitors and district nurses. However, in sexual health the term 'primary care' has an extended meaning, covering open access provision such as community contraceptive clinics, GUM and pharmacies. This book has been written for those who work in general practice and its associated health care team and so we have used primary care in its more restricted sense to signify this alone.

IMPORTANCE OF PRIMARY CARE

Sexual health is vital to overall health and wellbeing. Primary care has an enormous contribution to make to this area. The 2004 contract and the introduction of practice based commissioning provide the basis for important developments and we hope that all those working in general practice will seize these opportunities to ensure that they meet the needs of those who seek their advice on sexual health in a sensitive, appropriate and effective way.

Chapter 1

PROFESSIONAL SKILL MIX

Catriona Sutherland, Shelley Mehigan and Caroline Davey

INTRODUCTION

This chapter considers how primary care practitioners can work with each other and with professionals across a range of settings, in order to deliver the best possible sexual health services to patients. It begins by looking at how professional co-operation has evolved since the earliest days of family planning, and then goes on to explore ways of enhancing professional skill mix in the light of the National Strategy for Sexual Health and HIV, the General Medical Services (GMS) contract, and the Public Health White Paper, *Choosing Health*[1]. The final part of the chapter looks at ways to shape services for the future.

HOW PROFESSIONAL COOPERATION HAS EVOLVED

The past

Professional skill mix has been used in the delivery of sexual health services since the earliest days. When Marie Stopes set up the first family planning clinic in 1921, the original staff were a qualified midwife and a female doctor[2]. By 1924, 'instruction in the most satisfactory method of contraception' was given by registered medical practitioners assisted by qualified nurses[3]. During the 1930s, training provided by the National Birth Control Association (NBCA) was extended to include midwives, nurses and local authority doctors. The association changed its name in 1939 to the Family Planning Association (FPA), now **fpa**. During the war, the FPA's family clinics were largely run by nurses because of the lack of doctors.

In the early days of the NHS, there were arguments between general practitioners and the Ministry of Health about giving contraceptive advice free. By 1966, many more professionals, including health visitors, midwives, home nurses and social workers, were being encouraged to give family planning advice as part of their daily work. GPs provided most of the often limited contraceptive advice themselves at this time. Some areas ran a domiciliary service supported by health authorities and the FPA.

In 1975, GPs agreed to provide contraception as part of NHS services, but refused to supply free condoms to men on the grounds that they were non-medical devices. A number of GPs at this time were undergoing training with the FPA.

As far back as 1976, a Department of Health and Social Security working group recommended that, in addition to doctors, suitably trained nurses, midwives, health visitors, and some pharmacists, should be able to prescribe the contraceptive pill, to make it easier to access[4].

By the 1980s, some GPs were referring their patients to gynaecologists or local family planning clinics for services that they could not provide in their practice. A few practices employed family planning trained nurses to work with GPs in providing dedicated family planning sessions. Increasingly cervical screening was also included in family planning.

The position today

The training available to nurses and doctors has altered and expanded to reflect the huge changes that have taken place. Now that family planning is considered to be part of reproductive and sexual health, clients are able to receive holistic care throughout their reproductive and sexual lives. By the end of the 1990s, most nurses undertaking family planning training were working in general practice, many GPs had a keen interest in the subject, and around 75 per cent of contraceptive care was provided in general practice.

There were further developments in 2002, when the National Chlamydia Screening Programme was launched following high rates of chlamydia being identified, particularly among young people. This opportunistic screening programme is being delivered across a range of settings including general practice. It was initially implemented in ten areas, but now covers over 25 per cent of primary care trusts (PCTs) in England, and will be rolled out across England by March 2007. The programme has provided a key opportunity for both doctors and nurses working in primary care to improve their skills in this area and to get more involved in the delivery of sexual health services.

On 1 April 2004, the GMS contract was launched. This restructured the way that general practices operated and introduced three levels of services: essential, additional, and enhanced services. In theory, this clarifies what general practices provide, for example essential services should include sexual history-taking, consultations about sexually transmissible infections (STIs), HIV, unwanted pregnancy, and referral to other services such as genitourinary medicine (GUM) or abortion services. In addition, those practices which sign up to provide contraception as an additional service are required to give advice about the full range of methods. However, anecdotal evidence indicates that services available from practices still vary widely, with some practices interpreting the provisions of the 2004 contract – particularly regarding essential services – more narrowly than others.

In some areas, facilitators are visiting practices to run workshops for all interested members of the primary health care team (PHCT). Issues covered included confidentiality, access, teaching condom use and sexual history-taking.

The way forward

Key developments have taken place in primary care following the launch of the National Strategy for Sexual Health and HIV[5]. These include not only the significant changes that have taken place as part of the 2004 GMS contract but also the drivers in the Public Health White Paper for primary care taking a greater role in the provision of sexual health services. The White Paper proposes that services should be provided by a 'flexible, multidisciplinary workforce in a range of settings', and makes particular reference to:

- multidisciplinary teams headed by nurses
- extension of the roles of nurses
- mainstream primary care health programmes delivered by, among others, practice nurses
- 'enhanced services' in the new primary medical care contracts
- more 'primary care practitioners with a special interest' working alongside sexual health experts in contraceptive, HIV and sexual health treatment services.

With the increased profile given to the delivery of sexual health services in primary care, there is significant scope for doctors, nurses and ancillary staff to develop their skills in this area through the 'practitioners with special interest' route. Specific guidance exists for GPs with a special interest in sexual health, as well as for nurses and allied health professionals with special interests. These specialisms will also integrate well with the provision of enhanced services through the GMS contract.

Specifically, there are two national enhanced services which relate to sexual health – IUDs, and More Specialised Sexual Health Services. In addition, PCTs can choose to develop local enhanced services including expanding the provision of implants, developing young people's sexual health services, and extending training programmes to provide Level One services as defined by the National Strategy for Sexual Health and HIV.

What now happens in practice will depend on a number of factors, including national and local priorities, practice personnel, effective team work, resources, support and training. Below we consider how some of these areas can be addressed.

TEAMWORKING

What is needed to create an effective team?

Effective team working can only be achieved by all members knowing what others can do, and when, where and how they can be accessed. Appropriate support and training are also essential.

Support can be achieved by:

- clinical supervision
- debriefing after sessions or following critical incidents
- regular whole team meetings
- networks.

Training should always be relevant both to the practice and to individual team members, and should cover areas such as:

- confidentiality and consent, child protection, access to services, access to emergency contraception (EC) and condom supply mechanisms for the whole team
- STI courses for doctors, nurses and health advisers
- supply of emergency contraception by nurses and health advisers
- contraception training for doctors and nurses
- some nurses training to carry out procedures previously only performed by doctors (implant, IUD, IUS)
- cervical screening training for doctors and nurses
- sexual dysfunction and pregnancy counselling for clinicians and counsellors
- independent and supplementary nurse prescribing.

Ideally, the teaching of many of these topics should be delivered in an integrated way, so that, for example, clinicians link chlamydia testing with provision of emergency contraception wherever it is appropriate.

fpa and NHS Direct also play a part in providing information and training for professionals, as well as information and advice for the public.

How teams evolve

A primary care team may evolve in a way that is unplanned, planned, or in response to a critical incident. It may evolve in an unplanned way by incidentally employing someone who happens to have training, experience or interest in this area. This person then drives forward the development of the service.

The team may evolve in a planned way through internal or external forces.

- **Internal forces**: this may be as part of the whole philosophy of the practice and may include employing those who have already undertaken the relevant training, and developing training and education for the whole team.

- **External forces**: this may be as a response to:
    - national policies such as the Sexual Health Strategy
    - PCT policies
    - local public health concerns
    - stories in the media
    - individuals, for example, school nurse, youth worker, client/community demand
    - identified local needs.

The team may also evolve due to a critical incident. This may trigger the need to develop a practice protocol to guide future activities. For example, a receptionist carries out a pregnancy test on a sample brought in by a patient. It is only when the result is unexpected that the implications of dealing with the situation arise.

HOW SKILL MIX MIGHT WORK

Within all teams, whatever their size, skill mix is present to some degree.

Skill mix can be vertical, horizontal or parallel. The examples below identify models for a range of settings for sexual health and family planning services. Members of the team and the skills that they offer are also listed.

General practice with a special interest in sexual health

This general practice has a large pool of health care professionals, many highly trained in family planning and STIs. They include:

- eight GPs, two sessional GPs and two GP registrars
- one nurse practitioner and independent prescriber
- five practice nurses (three family planning trained, one of whom is an independent prescriber, and four STI-trained)
- two health advisers.

Between them, they offer a full range of contraceptive methods, including insertion and removal of implants, and insertion of intrauterine devices and systems (IUD and IUS); sexual health screening and management of some STIs, partner notification, pre-test counselling, hepatitis B immunisation, condom supply, pregnancy testing, pregnancy counselling, sexual dysfunction, cervical screening and EC.

Specialist young people's services

In this service, everyone has received some sexual health training and all staff have a special interest in young people. The team includes:

- three GPs, all contraception-trained and two STI-trained
- two nurses, both contraception-trained, one GUM-trained and the other STI-trained
- youth adviser who is STI-trained
- receptionist with a special interest in young people
- access to two counsellors, both with an interest in young people
- regular input from teenage pregnancy adviser, Connexions (an information and advice service for 13–19 year olds living in England)
- occasional input from health visitor, midwife and school liaison youth worker.

Large inner city practice

There is a whole-practice approach to the provision of sexual health services.

All personnel have received some sexual health training relevant to their role and many are highly trained. The team includes:

- eight GPs, two registrars
- five nurses, one nurse practitioner, one of the nurses is an independent prescriber

- two health advisers
- one health care assistant
- two sexual health outreach workers (who visit parenting groups, schools, youth groups, homeless hostels).

Sexual health service

This is a fully integrated sexual health service combining infection, contraception, HIV and sexual health promotion services. Clinics in all fields run alongside each other, with all personnel receiving a minimum of basic education in fields outside their own area of expertise. Some have more than one area of expertise. They include:

- a service manager, a clinical admin manager, an IT manager
- consultants in GUM, family planning and HIV, specialist registrars, GP registrars, two clinical assistants, sessional GPs
- three clinical nurse specialists, ten nurses, sexual health liaison nurse
- three health advisers, three healthcare assistants, one medical laboratory scientific officer
- reception and administrative staff
- a health promotion team.

NHS walk-in centre

This is facilitated by the local PCT and staffed by nurse practitioners who are able to issue EC using patient group directions (see page 31). The training that the nurses undergo is devised for them in conjunction with the sexual health clinic and the PCT pharmacy adviser.

Rural practice

The practice is sited in a village with a community sixth form college. The village draws young people from surrounding villages in an area with poor transport links. The need had been identified locally to tackle increasing rates of STIs and teenage pregnancy. There is now an innovative service:

- the GP runs a 'surgery' at the college during the lunch break once every two weeks, alternating with
- the practice nurse who is trained in contraception and sexual health and has a particular interest in young people, and

- the school nurse who is trained to issue EC under patient group directions.

Urban practice

The practice has two male GPs. One of the two practice nurses is a contraceptive specialist nurse. The local PCT identifies a need for this expertise to be available in other practices. A scheme is developed to fund the nurse to work sessions in neighbouring practices.

Skills and knowledge for clinicians in primary care

General, for all clinical staff

- Confidentiality for under-16s (see Fraser Guidance, Chapter 5, page 141, and Department of Health guidance for health professionals on treating under 16s[6]).
- Confidentiality.
- Routes of access to all aspects of care (whether provided 'in house' or not).

Specific clinical skills for some or all clinical team members

Sexual history/sexual health promotion

- Sexual history and risk assessment.
- Individual advice and sexual health promotion.

Prescribing

- Appropriate prescribing according to current guidance.

Cervical cytology

- Effective supervision of cervical cytology call, recall, follow-up and audit systems.
- Advice on the prevention of cervical cancer.
- Taking a cervical smear.

Contraceptive services

- Contraceptive advice on selection and use of the full range of methods.
- Provision of oral, patch and injectable hormonal contraception.
- Provision of emergency contraception.
- IUD fitting and removal*.
- Contraceptive implant fitting and removal*.
- Pre-abortion discussion and follow-up*.

STI services

- STI testing and associated discussion:
  - for men*
  - for women
  - on urine, swab, blood or other samples as appropriate
  - including HIV
  - interpretation of results.
- Knowledge of management principles of STIs including:
  - treatment of STIs
  - partner notification: awareness of current guidance
  - need to offer tests for some STIs (for example, chlamydia and HIV) when another STI is diagnosed.

Practices with particular expertise

- Conducting partner notification in collaboration with local services.
- Local and community approaches to education in sexual health.

*Some practices may not be able to provide these services, in which case signposting for access to care should be excellent, and onward referral high quality and fast.

HOW IT CAN WORK IN PRACTICE

Below, a series of scenarios outline a patient's typical journey across a range of services, and identify what the patient's experience of that service might be. The final scenario gives a vision of how effective skill mix across professions might improve access to services in the future.

The whole practice

M, a 19-year-old young man, sees the practice nurse for a new patient check, during which it becomes clear that he has symptoms of what may be an STI. The nurse discusses the options open to M and arranges for him to have some tests taken at that time. The nurse also offers him the opportunity to discuss sexual health issues with the sexual health worker who has a particular remit to promote good sexual health practices among young men. When M returns for his results with the GP registrar, he is also able to see the sexual health adviser to discuss issues.

Patient experience: any one member of the team may be able to fulfil some or all sexual health needs.

Multi-agency approach

C, a 24 year old woman, visits the NHS walk-in centre requesting the emergency contraceptive pill. After discussing the options with the nurse, C decides she would like to have an emergency contraception IUD. The walk-in centre nurse calls through to the sexual health clinic to check availability of appointments and gives C a referral note to take with her to the clinic the next day. In accordance with the Faculty of Family Planning and Reproductive Health Care guidelines she is given Levonelle ®2 anyway, in case she is unable to attend for the fitting. C is seen the next day in the IUD clinic, where she is counselled, screened for STIs, treated prophylactically because of the identified risk of an STI, and fitted with an emergency IUD. She is given information regarding ongoing contraception as she wishes to consider her options. She will return to discuss this when she comes back to have the IUD removed. She also knows that she can return at any time if she is concerned.

Patient experience: co-ordinated working between different teams in different settings ensures the patient gets the service she wants.

Specialist young people's services

T, a 17-year-old young woman, sees the nurse following treatment for a second STI. There is discussion about the infection, about her relationship, and her feelings to do with trying to assert herself with condom use. She then reveals that she has 'a lot of stress' and that she tries to cope with this by cutting herself. She is frightening herself and her close friends and wants some help. The youth worker is free at that time and T agrees to see him. He makes an initial assessment and has many concerns about her. T agrees to wait and see the doctor. She is prescribed medication and agrees to see the youth worker or counsellor on a weekly basis.

Patient experience: dedicated, holistic, weekly walk-in session for all aged 13–19 years, provided by a regular, small team. Patients can see all or any of the team members, depending on their needs on that day.

The future: professional skill mix

S visits her local pharmacy to pick up a repeat supply of her contraceptive pills. She is taking a combined contraceptive pill. The pharmacist has completed the training to become a supplementary prescriber and is working to a patient care management plan formulated with S's GP. Both the pharmacist and the GP undertook the supplementary prescriber training at the local university, where they also met clinicians from the local sexual health clinic. The GP and pharmacist are kept up-to-date with new developments in the field of contraception electronically by regular mailings and via the clinic website.

As part of the consultation the pharmacist identifies that S has suffered two attacks of migraine since her last visit. He refers S back to her general practice for an appointment with the practice nurse who has a special interest in contraception. In case S is unable to get an appointment before she runs out of pills he also gives her the contact details for the sexual health clinic. The pharmacist is confident that these details are up-to-date as he is in regular contact with the sexual health community liaison nurse. The clinic organises annual updates for GPs, nurses and pharmacists.

Patient experience: much improved access to co-operative and co-ordinated services in her community

Primary care based sexual health outreach worker (SHOW) project

A practice in an urban deprived area has a list size of 7,500 patients. Sexual health problems are common, including high rates of unwanted pregnancy, chlamydia and HIV.

As a personal medical services (PMS) practice, funding was sought for an integrated approach to sexual health. Funding was originally obtained from a community health trust, a primary care group (PCG) and a community regeneration organisation. Two sexual health workers were employed to work with both the lead practice and also four neighbouring practices in what became known as the SHOW project.

One worker (non-clinical) was male with a background in sexual health promotion with socially excluded young men. After being appointed to the practice, he gained skills in discussion of STI tests and in phlebotomy. He also gained knowledge of how care is accessed in primary care; and partner notification, and increased his factual knowledge in contraception and STIs and their management. Shortly he will be learning how to take urethral swabs from men, until full urine testing is available locally.

The other worker (clinical) was female, with a background in health advising and practice nursing. After being appointed to the practice she consolidated her clinical skills in contraceptive care and STI diagnosis. She learned to manage women with unwanted pregnancy for referral on for fast track abortion services when appropriate. She obtained the NHS cervical screening certificate. She is now able to fit contraceptive implants and also IUDs. She has developed skills in education to support development work with the participating practices. It is hoped she will become a nurse prescriber in due course.

The SHOWs provide contraceptive care with active follow-up, condoms, STI testing, partner notification, fast track abortion referral and sexual health promotion as appropriate. The clinical worker will co-ordinate treatment for STIs (still prescribed by the GPs). Outreach community prevention work (led by the non-clinical worker) with local young people, and also with community workers, delivers sexual health promotion, and also aims to improve access to care.

Both SHOWs work collaboratively with each other, with the primary care teams, and with local services (including the labs). Clinical staff at participating practices are taught how to use risk assessment in order to identify those patients at highest risk for face-to-face work with one of the sexual health workers.

The project is now in its fifth year, and is funded directly by the PCT – although it is still managed and housed by the lead practice.

SUPPLYING MEDICINES TO PATIENTS

The advent of nurse prescribing and greater skill mix has meant that supplying medicines is now more complicated. It was becoming increasingly common for a practice nurse who had trained in family planning (along with those trained in other specialised areas) to 'advise' his or her GPs what was the most up-to-date thinking and which pills were most frequently and appropriately prescribed in clinics. This is likely to have been one of the many triggers for the situation that was finally resolved by the Crown reviews.

REVIEWS OF THE MEDICINES ACT

The Medicines Act of 1968 allowed for appropriate practitioners to be able to prescribe medicines. Initially these practitioners were doctors, dentists and vets, but the Act was written in a way that allowed for amendment by statutory instrument. Following the Cumberlege Report of 1986[7], Dr June Crown[8] chaired her first review of the Act. As a result, the Act was extended to include nurses, although it was limited to nurses who had completed health visitor or district nurse training, and only related to items such as dressings and appliances likely to be used by community nurses. In 1997, Professor June Crown chaired a further review looking at all aspects of prescribing, supply and administration of medicines, including the use of protocols.

Recommendations on use of protocols

Use of protocols had arisen out of a desire to improve access for patients to supplies of medication. The Medicines Act allowed for the supplying and administering of medicines to be delegated to appropriately trained nurses in certain circumstances. The legality of protocols had not been tested and varying legal views were given over a period of time which left nurses and doctors uncertain of where they stood.

The Crown reviews[9,10] recommended three layers of prescribing: independent prescribing, dependent prescribing, and group protocols for the supply and administration to previously unidentified groups. After further consultation, the Department of Health announced a slightly amended version of these, namely:

- **Independent prescribing**: these are nurses (and possibly others) who can prescribe in their own right using individual prescription pads from an extended but still limited formulary.

- **Supplementary prescribing**: nurses and pharmacists (and possibly others) who can prescribe on an individual prescription pad *any* medicine in the British National Formulary (BNF) according to a patient care management plan devised in conjunction with a doctor for an individual patient.

- **Patient group directions (PGDs)**: these allow for the supply of one-off medicines to previously unidentified groups of patients, for example, immunisations, travel vaccines and emergency contraception.

At the time of going to print, the Department of Health was in the process of reviewing this area, and is likely to increase independent prescribing by extended formulary nurse prescribers in the future.

Improving access to contraceptive services for patients

The prescribing measures outlined above provide the basis on which we can now build our services for the future. It enables clinicians to take responsibility for their own decisions and for the most appropriate clinician to offer a particular service.

- Some pharmacists, school nurses, A&E nurses and nurses in NHS walk-in centres can supply emergency contraception using PGDs.

- Nurses and pharmacists are able to undertake supplementary prescribing according to patient care management plans.

- Independent nurse prescribers are able to prescribe those products which are on the extended formulary.

- Pharmacists can sell the pharmacy version of emergency contraception to those who are 16 or over.

- In the future, pharmacists may be able to dispense repeat supplies of certain medicines and this may include contraceptive pills.

THE FUTURE

So what will the skill mix of the future look like? With the many recent developments in the sexual health field, there is huge potential to create services that truly respond to identified needs using a much wider group of professionals. It is anticipated that there will be more nurse-led work and an increased role for non-medical staff. Training is one area that is likely to become multidisciplinary sooner rather than later. Already, in a few areas, nurses and pharmacists are undertaking supplementary prescribing courses. It also makes sense for doctors and nurses to train together in the field of sexual health. As the emphasis moves toward more experiential learning, specialist nurses should increasingly be recognised as appropriate trainers of doctors.

Key messages

Skill mix:

- is a way of improving access to services, and providing a more appropriate range of services
- offers a more efficient and appropriate use of staff and skills
- enhances skills and personal development
- fills previously unmet needs in that setting.

References

1. Department of Health. *National Strategy for Sexual Health and HIV*. London: Department of Health 2001; Department of Health. *Standard General Medical Services Contract.* Department of Health 2004; Department of Health. *Choosing Health: Making healthy choices easier.* London: The Stationery Office 2004.

2. Leathard A. *The Fight for Family Planning* Chap 1. London: Macmillan 1980.

3. Leathard A. *The Fight for Family Planning* Chap 4. London: Macmillan 1980.

4. Department of Health and Social Security. *Report of the Joint Working Group on Oral Contraceptives*. London: HMSO 1976.

5. See note 1 above.

6. *Best Practice Guidance for Doctors and Other Health Professionals on the Provision of Advice and Treatment to Young People Under 16 on Contraception, Sexual and Reproductive Health.* London: Department of Health 2004.

7. Department of Health and Social Security. *Neighbourhood Nursing: A Focus for Care*. London: HMSO 1986.

8. Department of Health. *Report of the Advisory Group on Nurse Prescribing.* London: Department of Health 1989.

9. Department of Health. *A Report on the Supply and Administration of Medicines Under Group Protocols*. London: Department of Health 1998.

10. Department of Health. *Review of Prescribing, Supply and Administration of Medicines. Final Report (Crown 11 Report)*. London: Department of Health 1999.

Diagram 1.1 How skill mix works in practice

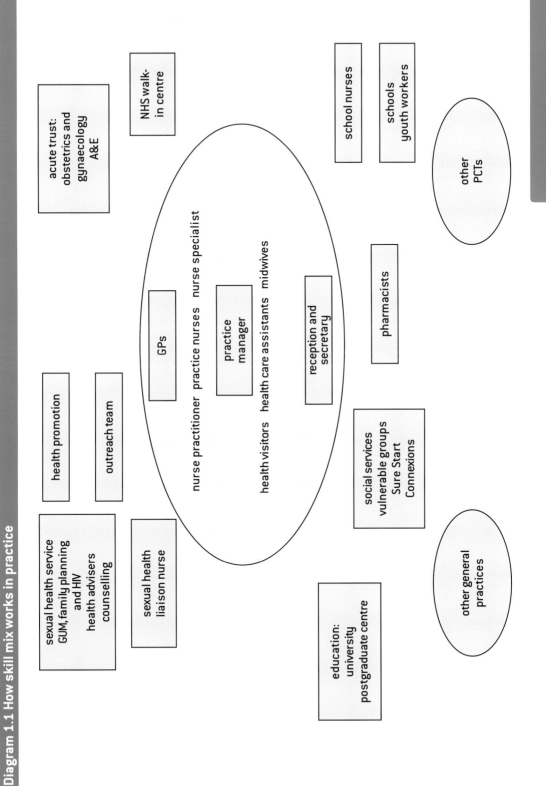

acute trust:
obstetrics and
gynaecology
A&E

NHS walk-
in centre

school nurses

schools
youth workers

other
PCTs

health promotion

outreach team

nurse practitioner practice nurses nurse specialist

GPs

practice
manager

health visitors health care assistants midwives

reception and
secretary

pharmacists

sexual health service
GUM, family planning
and HIV
health advisers
counselling

sexual health
liaison nurse

social services
vulnerable groups
Sure Start
Connexions

education:
university
postgraduate centre

other general
practices

Chapter 2

RISK ASSESSMENT AND SEXUAL HISTORY-TAKING IN PRIMARY CARE

Philippa Matthews and Rita Ireson

INTRODUCTION

The cornerstone of effective sexual health services in primary care is the clinician's ability to identify which patients, of the many they see, are at risk of an unplanned pregnancy or sexually transmissible infection (STI). This is not a simple matter of a 'one-size-fits-all' approach. The diversity of patients we see in primary care means that we need a clear process for assessing risk relatively quickly, and in a way that is meaningful to the patient. We fail those patients who *are* at risk if we are unable to identify who they are; we do a disservice to those patients who are *not* at risk if we inappropriately target them with unnecessary sexual health interventions.

Assessment of risk of sexual ill health is not a precise science. It has two important aspects which relate to 'risk groups' and 'risk behaviour' – two useful terms that should not be confused.

- Knowledge of groups at higher risk (that is, a higher than 'average' risk) – for example: young people; those with a recent history of abortion; a history of STI; or those from countries with a high prevalence of HIV. Use of this 'risk group' concept *may* help prioritise those patients from whom you take a sexual history. However, responding to an individual in a risk group should not lead to inappropriate assumptions about their individual risk.

- Sexual history-taking – informs the assessment of an individual's risk of unplanned pregnancy or an STI. This mainly centres on risk *behaviours*: partner history, condom use, sexual practices and contraceptive use. A clinical judgment is then made on the basis of this and other information or knowledge that you have of the patient.

It is not only the clinician who may gain useful information by taking a sexual history. The process of history-taking can also be informative for the patient. It often makes clear why the doctor or nurse is – or is not – concerned about the patient's risk of having a sexual health problem. It clarifies the routes by which STIs are transmitted and how long infections may be present. The process of history-taking also emphasises that infections can be present without symptoms. A careful assessment of contraceptive use (for those methods that are user-dependent) may also highlight any misunderstandings that the patient has about how to use her or his contraceptive method.

Sexual history-taking is also important when assessing sexual dysfunction. Sexual problems and sexual dysfunction are discussed more fully in Chapter 8.

Clinicians need to take an integrated and flexible approach to sexual history-taking so that they can give appropriate emphasis for each consultation. This chapter, of necessity, focuses on the clinician's agenda, and aims to demonstrate the value of sexual history-taking as a clinical tool. While not addressed to the same degree here, there is enormous value in those aspects of a consultation that are patient-led and which centre on the patient's own agenda. The clinician's excellent listening and communication skills will underpin all effective sexual history-taking, regardless of whose agenda is to fore.

This chapter offers a comprehensive, step-by-step guide to taking a sexual history, including practical advice on all aspects of the process: partner history, condom use, sexual practices and contraceptive use. It initially explores why and when to take a sexual history, and then offers ideas about how to take a sexual history in primary care.

WHY USE RISK ASSESSMENT IN PRIMARY CARE?

Unmet need
Sexual health in primary care is characterised by unrecognised and unmet need. STIs are increasingly common. They can be asymptomatic or only subtly symptomatic (see Chapter 6). Ninety-three per cent of teenagers who go on to have a pregnancy have consulted in primary care in the preceding year. Of these, 71 per cent had consultations about contraception[1]. Around 9–10 per cent of sexually active young women using primary care will have chlamydia infection[2]. Sixty-five per cent of women with HIV consulted in primary care in the year before diagnosis[3]. One study of 71 street-based prostitutes found that GPs were the main source of all types of health care, with frequent attendance[4].

It is thought that about a third of HIV infection in the UK is undiagnosed – with heterosexual HIV over-represented in the undiagnosed group[5]. Some of these patients may have their sexual health issue as a 'hidden agenda' when they attend. However, in many of these instances, the patient may have no real sense that they are at risk of unplanned pregnancy, chlamydia, or HIV – or perhaps all three.

Primary care service users come from across the spectrum of risk

Genitourinary medicine (GUM) clinics see individuals at particularly high risk of STIs[6]. In the GUM context, it is good practice to offer *all* attenders tests for chlamydia and HIV. In primary care, on the other hand, we see people from across the spectrum of risk of sexual health problems. Our service users may have high risk for STIs, or have no risk at all. It is neither feasible nor appropriate in primary care to discuss HIV or chlamydia tests with *all* attenders; instead, we have to adopt a range of approaches.

Risk groups and risk behaviour

Awareness of which groups are at highest risk of a health problem can help target interventions. For example, most new HIV infection acquired in the UK is still in men who have sex with men. Prevention and detection strategies should, quite appropriately, prioritise this group, using outreach work and other strategies. Nevertheless, there are many gay men who, for a variety of reasons, are at no risk at all of HIV. In the same way, international travellers as a group are at risk of acquiring STIs abroad, yet many individual travellers may be at no risk whatsoever. Primary care can respond to knowledge about risk groups (for example, by setting up a young people's clinic), but sexual history-taking is also needed in order to assess *individual* risk.

Risk indicators which are relevant to primary care

There are a number of factors associated with risky sexual behaviour and sexual health problems:

How different aspects of sexual health interrelate

Associations between different aspects of sexual ill-health are now well recognised. Risk of unplanned pregnancy or STIs appears to be associated with:

- past history of STI within recent years
- past history of abortion within recent years

- recent or multiple use of emergency contraception – and possibly chaotic use of contraception – (associated with risk of unplanned pregnancy).

In addition:

- some strains of human papilloma virus (HPV) infection are associated with increased risk of cervical cancer
- patients with one STI are commonly found to have another
- the presence of almost any STI is associated with increased risk of transmission of HIV, if the patient is sexually exposed to this.

Other health issues linked with sexual ill-health

- mental health problems
- drug misuse and alcohol problems
- smoking (associated with an increased risk of cervical cancer)
- women at highest risk of cervical cancer may be more likely to remain unscreened: this may reflect limited health-seeking behaviour.

'Social exclusion' issues associated with sexual health problems

The under-25s are at increased risk of having an unplanned pregnancy or STI, but within this group there are young people at especially high risk. These are young people:

- with low educational attainment/poor negotiation skills
- who are within the public care system
- who are from a single-parent family.

Specific issues associated with risk

- those who have recently had a change of partner – for example, recently divorced or separated
- those who come from countries with a higher prevalence of HIV may reflect the same level of prevalence in their UK-based communities.

Use of risk indicators in primary care

Risk factors are more or less visible to us. Our records tell us that a patient is a teenager before they enter the consulting room. However, we may or may not have any indication that they binge-drink alcohol at the weekends. We may well remain unaware of which men are gay, let alone which gay men are at risk of HIV[7].

A 35-year old woman recorded as married does not belong to a group which is apparently a high priority for sexual health care – unless, for example, she works in the sex industry, or her husband regularly buys unprotected sex. There will always be factors that may be highly relevant to clinical care that nevertheless remain invisible to us. However, risk assessment and sexual history-taking can be valuable in identifying risk factors, and so can help to support clinical decision-making.

Those at no risk

'Everyone is at risk of having a sexually transmissible infection' is a useful working assumption in a GUM clinic, but patently untrue in primary care. Taking an approach that assumes everyone is at risk causes offence, and also confuses messages about how to keep safe. GPs and practice nurses may not be certain who is and who is not at risk – but they need pragmatic strategies for dealing with patients who are at *no apparent* risk.

WHY AND WHEN TO USE SEXUAL HISTORY-TAKING

There are a number of situations during consultations with a patient when taking a sexual history can be a great help. These are summarised below, and then explored individually in more depth.

Sexual history-taking helps in the process of diagnosing and managing STIs:

- to aid in the process of differential diagnosis (see also Chapter 6)
- to decide whether a test for an STI is appropriate
- to obtain informed consent for STI tests
- to help interpret STI test results.

Sexual history-taking helps to inform contraceptive care:

- by identifying who might benefit from more proactive contraceptive follow-up
- by identifying who might benefit from a shift to less 'user-dependent' contraceptive methods
- by promoting condom use in a targeted way
- by choosing a contraceptive method appropriate to a woman's risk of STI.

Sexual history-taking helps in the promotion of sexual health:

- by identifying which patients need advice – and which do not
- by enabling sexual health advice to be tailored to individual patients.

Sexual history-taking to support the process of differential diagnosis

The symptoms and signs that STIs may present in primary care are covered in Chapter 6. Many of these symptoms can have other possible causes. GPs need the clinical knowledge to know when an STI might be a cause – but once this has been indicated, they cannot simply refer *all* patients with these symptoms to GUM. Doing a risk assessment with the patient will help the GP to establish how likely it is that an STI is the cause. Is it likely that a 6-week old baby's sticky eye is due to chlamydia? Could the patient's weight loss and persistent diarrhoea be due to HIV? Are those genital ulcers due to herpes or Behcets? These are the kinds of situation in which risk assessment can help to save time and guide investigation and referral.

Sexual history-taking to decide whether a test for an STI is appropriate

As discussed above, with symptomatic patients a risk assessment for STI will guide decisions to offer tests. Risk assessment can also be very helpful with *asymptomatic* patients. Some patients may request tests, but a risk assessment will establish if they are at no risk of an STI, and instead simply require advice and reassurance. People who have many changes of partner – particularly men who have sex with men – are at increased risk of hepatitis B, and should be offered a test to check immunity. Those at very high risk of hepatitis B might be offered the first immunisation at the same time (see Chapter 6).

Sexual history-taking to obtain informed consent for STI tests

The process of doing a risk assessment for STI with a patient will in itself help the patient to understand why a test is – or is not – indicated. This is a very good basis for gaining informed consent to a test.

Sexual history-taking to help interpret STI test results

Knowledge of the test used, coupled with knowledge of the history, helps in the interpretation of test results – particularly negative results. (False positives are now less of a problem, because of the improvement in available tests.)

Sexual history-taking to identify who might benefit from more proactive contraceptive follow-up, and to identify who might benefit from a shift to less 'user-dependent' contraceptive methods

A careful assessment of contraceptive use is important with patients on user-dependent methods, such as oral contraception or contraceptive patches. Some patients may follow instructions closely, and so there is little extra contraceptive cover to be gained by a switch to less user-dependent methods. However, one study of teenagers who became pregnant found that 65 per cent had obtained the combined oral contraceptive pill from primary care in the year preceding the pregnancy[8]. This may be because this contraceptive method is not suitable for this group, or that the information and support offered were inadequate. A thorough history of contraceptive use and beliefs can be illuminating for clinicians as well as for the patient. We should also bear in mind associations with unplanned pregnancy (such as young age and social exclusion).

Sexual history-taking to promote condom use in a targeted way

Across-the-board advice to all patients to use condoms may not engage individual patients to change their practice – especially if they do not perceive themselves to be at risk, or if they do not think that the advice applies to them. Assessing risk for STI and unplanned pregnancy may bring home the issues to individuals and help to motivate change.

Sexual history-taking to choose a contraceptive method appropriate to a woman's risk of STI

Current risk of STI indicates whether a chlamydia test is required, especially if an intrauterine device (IUD) is to be fitted. Possible future risk should be discussed with some patients when looking at contraceptive choice, because it will highlight the need to consider use of condoms. Future risk may also influence choices about non-barrier methods (most notably, but not solely, IUDs).

Sexual history-taking to target who does – or does not – need advice, and to tailor sexual health advice to individual patients

Sexual history-taking can quite quickly help us to assess risk, so that sexual health promotion advice can focus on those who need it. Not all international travellers will be exposed to risk of HIV or hepatitis B; time may be better spent discussing sun protection. It is not a priority for all women attending for smears to be given advice about how to protect their sexual health and reduce risk of cervical cancer in the future. Some users of oral contraception can readily understand the use of emergency contraception if pills are missed; some need more time and information about when to seek advice. In all these situations, a good risk assessment can identify who needs advice, and what advice is most appropriate – thus increasing its relevance to the individual patient.

Joining up the history

Clearly, many of the areas identified above interrelate. It is important to have an integrated model of the sexual history so that all the relevant aspects of sexual health can be addressed. It is all too easy to practise in a particular sub-section of sexual health (*'This is a consultation on contraception – I will use my contraceptive and menstrual histories'*) and totally overlook the other – related – aspects of sexual health. A joined-up sexual history can bring together the artificially fragmented components of sexual health into a more meaningful and realistic whole.

SEXUAL HISTORY-TAKING IN PRIMARY CARE

Confidentiality

If a patient does not feel that their care is confidential, then quality of care is compromised and the patient will not feel able to discuss their sexual history. It is very important that patients are made aware that a practice takes confidentiality seriously. The rights of young people to confidential care need to be well understood by all team members. Clinical staff should be familiar with and able to apply Fraser Guidance (see page 141). As well as other key aspects of confidentiality (discussed in detail in Chapter 5), sexual history-taking should not be conducted where the consultation can be overheard (for example, behind a curtain).

Communication

It is not possible to teach communication skills in one chapter of a book. However, some aspects are particularly important for sexual history-taking. Excellent listening skills are assumed.

Being able to respond to hidden agendas and important disclosures

Sexual history-taking can lead to important disclosures. Taking a partner history or asking about condom use may lead the patient to think about highly personal issues – such as non-consensual sex, or erectile dysfunction. Clinicians who use such areas of questioning on a routine basis should always remain sensitive to how they ask questions. They should be highly alert to shifts in the patient's verbal and non-verbal responses which may signal distress and a need to create 'space' for the patient to share – or withhold – information that is highly personal. In these circumstances, the agenda of the clinician should be put on hold.

Clinicians need to be able to use both open and closed questions to take sexual histories. This chapter gives numerous examples of questions which are valuable in clinical practice – many of these are closed. The use of open questions is especially important when eliciting a hidden agenda, or when responding to a disclosure.

If a patient makes a disclosure of a traumatic experience – such as rape or childhood sexual abuse – the most important thing is to *listen*. The fact that the patient has chosen to tell this clinician – *you* – demonstrates that you are the right person. The patient will not expect you to have ready answers or crucial advice. If need be, arrange to meet again – and meanwhile, you can find out what advice or support is available.

Avoiding inappropriate assumptions

Assumptions save us time, and we do use them, quite appropriately, in the clinical context. Unfortunately, within the specific context of sexual history-taking, assumptions can cause problems. It may be reasonably safe to assume that a 32-year old woman who has come to renew her contraceptive diaphragm has, or intends to have, sex with a male partner. However, we cannot assume the same of a newly-registered 19-year old woman on the combined oral contraceptive pill – she might be using this to regulate her menstrual cycle.

When working with an individual from a 'risk' group in a consultation – for example, a gay man or a teenage girl – we cannot afford to make assumptions about the individual risks each might face. The gay man may be in a mutually monogamous relationship of 23 years' standing; the teenage girl might hold a strong religious belief that sex before marriage is unacceptable. This is our difficulty in primary care – if we wish to be proactive about sexual health with our service users, we must learn to approach such discussions without making assumptions. The degree to which we have to do this is unique amongst services providing sexual health care. Neither the gay man nor the teenager is likely to attend a specialist sexual health service – but they are both likely to attend primary care. However, we will *also* see the gay man at high risk of HIV and the teenager at high risk of unplanned pregnancy[9].

If a wrong assumption *is* made by a clinician, this can occasionally misdirect a whole consultation – for example, a lengthy recommendation to use contraception to a woman who has a female partner, or a warning to a young person about the risks of chlamydia when the young person has never had sex. Such assumptions can cause considerable offence to the patient, who may not return. However, if the clinician becomes aware of an erroneous assumption, it is best to be open and, if appropriate, to apologise. Patients will usually be quite pleased that the clinician has noticed the error and wants to make amends; this can even be a constructive step in the clinician/patient relationship.

Making judgements

A clinician may or may not feel disapproving of a patient's behaviours. Even the most tolerant among us is likely to encounter patients who have done something which we feel most uncomfortable about (even if we exclude consideration of the risk of harm to others, which might necessitate action). However, judgemental approaches can undermine our clinical ability. The skill is to conduct a history so that the patient feels free to give the information needed for clinical care, while still retaining trust in the clinician. Signalling a negative judgement can be avoided by focusing on the information that is needed for clinical purposes. *'Are you faithful?'* is a social, not a clinical question; *'Do you have any other sexual partners?'* is a clinical one. Patients making a disclosure may need reassurance that they are not being judged or blamed – for example, if they are in an abusive relationship or if they have sold sex.

Even carefully worded questions or reactions can convey judgement, depending on the intonation and delivery. Disapproval can also be transmitted non-verbally, through facial expressions and other body language. While this can all be explored through communication skills teaching, highly-motivated clinicians with good self-awareness may be able to identify, reflect upon and change their own judgemental behaviours.

Giving information

Information needs to be given in an ordered way that is appropriate to the understanding of the patient. The clinician should have familiar approaches to information-giving in a range of circumstances in order to ensure that no important points are missed. This can then be adapted to take into account the understanding of the patient. Standard information will need to be given in a large number of situations, including information on individual contraceptive methods, positive STI test results, smear taking, and discussion of smear results. Information often needs to be repeated, and will benefit from being backed-up with appropriate written information.

Giving results

Positive results – whether for an infection, pregnancy test or an abnormal smear – may come as a shock to the patient. It is best to give the result straight away to allow time to hear the patient and for discussion and explanation. In all circumstances, it is important to find positive and constructive information to contribute; the timing of this within the consultation will vary.

Checking understanding

In any communication with patients, the clinician may need to check that the patient has understood what has been said. However, within the context of a sexual history, the clinician, too, may not understand everything that is said by the patient, and so will need to check any words or phrases that they are unclear about.

Sexual problems and sexual dysfunction

Patients may present with, or disclose, sexual difficulties such as erectile dysfunction. Caring for patients with these problems is discussed in Chapter 8.

When sexual history-taking is difficult in primary care

There are a number of common circumstances in primary care that can make sexual history-taking difficult:

- the patient may not expect questions about sex
- the patient may not perceive him/herself to be at risk
- the patient may not be at risk
- there may be language and/or cultural differences
- the patient may be accompanied
- the clinician may be pressed for time
- the clinician may lack appropriate training and confidence.

Strategies for introducing the subject of sexual health when the patient doesn't expect questions about sex

GPs and practice nurses will find that they have to raise the subject of sexual health in a variety of clinical circumstances. The patient may or may not be expecting this. If a clinician moves directly to sexual history-taking, without explaining the clinical motivation for this, then the patient's mind may be racing to try to work out what on earth the clinician is up to. A young female student with a persistent mild conjunctivitis will be wondering why a male doctor is asking about sexual partners – she will not be in the best frame of mind to collaborate with the process of history-taking.

Strategies for introducing the subject of sexual health when the patient doesn't perceive that they are at risk

Our patients may not see themselves as being at risk, even when they are. Despite having 'traditional' STI symptoms such as vaginal discharge, patients may present in primary care without any sense that an STI could be a possibility for them. A range of beliefs can underpin this – commonly including a lack of understanding about how long some of the infections can be present, as well as a lack of knowledge about the asymptomatic nature of many infections. The clinician's job is to unfold the history with the patient, and to give relevant information, so that it is clear to the patient why they may be at risk.

Strategies for introducing the subject of sexual health when the patient is not at risk

We need to raise the subject of sexual health, but, after assessment, we may also need to drop it again, if the patient is at no apparent risk of a given (or any) sexual health problem. It is helpful in this situation if the clinician has managed to avoid assumptions from the outset.

Strategies for the patient with symptoms

One approach could be: *'There are a number of possible causes for your problem. One of these is – oddly enough – a sexually transmissible infection. Do you think you could be at risk? Could I ask you some questions so I can check?'* This kind of approach can be adapted to a whole range of circumstances, from possible neonatal conjunctivitis through to possible presentation with AIDS.

In the case of HIV, it may help to modify the introduction to indicate that this is a rare or remote possibility, but one that needs to be considered. [Having referred to other diagnostic possibilities]: *'There is a rare but serious cause for this that I need to consider, for the sake of completeness. Have you ever wondered if you could be at risk of HIV?'* Nothing can make this an easy interaction, but a doctor taking this approach is clinically safer than one in denial – and will often be met with considerable trust and openness by the patient.

Strategies for targeting sexual health promotion

Strategies for promoting sexual health in a range of scenarios are offered below:

'We find that young people in this area are at quite high risk of having sexually transmissible infections, so we like to raise this with all our newly-registered patients under 25. Could I ask you a few questions to see if you could be at risk?'

'You can see from this leaflet that you are travelling to an area with very high levels of sexually transmissible infections and HIV. Can I talk with you about whether you are likely to be at any risk or not?'

'There's no problem in you starting the pill, we can certainly arrange that. However, we find that we are seeing an increasing number of people with sexually

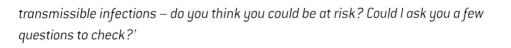

transmissible infections – do you think you could be at risk? Could I ask you a few questions to check?'

Dealing with language and cultural differences

Primary care is a service well-used by different ethnic groups – most notably women from all backgrounds. Sexual history-taking can be greatly compromised by language barriers, but is also one of the areas of enquiry in which reliance on a family member or friend to interpret is most inappropriate. Even the use of professional interpreters can pose difficulties if the interpreter and the patient are different genders, or if they are from the same small ethnic community. In addition, sex can be very difficult to discuss because of cultural differences between the clinician and the patient. There are no easy answers to these situations, which are an increasing part of our daily lives.

Strategies for dealing with the accompanied patient

In primary care, patients are often accompanied, sometimes by several people. Accompanying people may have been invited by the patient, or may be totally unwelcome.

- **Who is accompanying the patient?** This is best clarified if there is any uncertainty – we may know that a patient is a lesbian, but the woman accompanying her may be her friend, sister, partner or carer. Sometimes an introduction is volunteered, but if not, it is best actively to seek one: *'Hello, I am Dr Brown – I don't think we've met . . . ?' 'Sorry, I'm not quite clear – are you friends?' 'Is this your partner?'*

- **What is the content of the consultation?** If the consultation is going to be about whiplash, or a repeat emollient for eczema, it may not matter that the patient is accompanied. However, the content of the consultation will often not be apparent until it has started – possibly even to the patient, who has not thought that their symptoms might relate to sexual health. We need time to get the feel of the presenting (or subsequent) topics. Should a problem arise that may relate to sexual health (perhaps abdominal pain in a 24-year old), it is best to be quite directive: *'I'd now like to suggest that we talk alone for a moment –* [to accompanying person] *Would it be OK if you waited outside? You can rejoin us shortly.'* It is then possible to explain to the patient why you would like to take a sexual history. The patient can then choose whether the person outside the room is invited back in then, or later on.

- **Is the patient a young person accompanied by a parent or guardian?** This is sometimes to be welcomed, but can be a considerable hindrance: the difficulty lies in knowing which is the case in any given consultation. In general, it is not fair to ask the young person (in front of the parent) if they wish the adult to remain in the room, especially as the young person may not be anticipating that questioning about sexual health issues could arise. If a consultation may touch upon sexual health (for example, to check if oral contraceptives are being prescribed from elsewhere before an antibiotic is given), then it is appropriate for the doctor to take control and politely ask the adult to leave: '*At this practice we are trying to have a moment alone with anyone in this age group to chat over health issues.* [To parent] *Would it be possible for you to have a seat outside for a few minutes?*' You may wish to indicate that you will be inviting them to rejoin you in due course. This approach rarely leads to difficulties. After discussion with the young person about their right to confidential care, the parent can be invited straight back in if the young person wishes. If the young person prefers a private consultation, it is best to agree with them what will be said to the parent at the end of the consultation – whether the parent will be informed about all issues, or whether some agreed neutral topic will be introduced. If the young person does not wish to withhold any information from their parent at the end of the consultation, it may be constructive to point this out to the parent.

Strategies for dealing with a lack of time

With practice and experience, sexual history-taking does not take long with most patients. That minority of patients who require a significant amount of time are often those with high clinical need, so it is time well spent. Sexual history-taking can occasionally save time: if a woman with a vaginal discharge gives a history suggestive of vaginal candida and she is at no risk of having an STI, then there is no need to examine her or test for STIs (unless symptoms don't resolve with treatment). Similarly, a young woman with dysuria and frequency may be managed as though she has cystitis if she is at no risk of having an STI.

Strategies for dealing with a lack of training or confidence

Studies from the US suggest that patients find it difficult to raise the subject of sexual health and see it as the doctor's role to broach the subject. These findings may help to reassure GPs who are initially hesitant about raising the subject of sexual health with their patients. Confidence in sexual history-taking should grow with experience. In the early stages, GPs may find it helpful to use the actual phrases suggested in the section below. Finally, there are increasing opportunities for clinicians to access relevant teaching and training to improve skills.

This section focuses on key phrases to use when taking a sexual history. They have been tried and tested extensively, in real and simulated consultations, and in teaching situations. You may wish to adopt the phrases and use them verbatim; or to understand the underlying principles and then devise your own verbal strategies.

It is important to be clear in your own mind why taking a sexual history is clinically indicated (see *Why and when to use sexual history-taking*, page 39). This will help to focus on the relevant areas of questioning. A sexual history should *not* be taken until the patient understands the clinical reasons behind it (see *Strategies for introducing the subject of sexual health,* page 45 above). The patient is then more likely to be motivated to collaborate in the whole process: they will understand that it is in their own interest.

Sometimes clinicians are taking a sexual history to assess *current* risk of having an STI (for example, when assessing a patient with symptoms). Sometimes they need to assess *future* risk (for example, when a patient is about to go travelling abroad). Similarly, the future may be a key area of enquiry with a young person starting on contraception. It is important to be clear whether the focus for a given consultation is *risk to date* or *future risk* – or both.

Why systematic enquiries ('symptom questions') have limited value

When asked what a sexual history consists of, many clinicians imagine that it is a systematic enquiry relating to the reproductive system. However, given the diversity of possible symptoms of STIs, and the enormous burden of asymptomatic infection, this is often not a good use of time. Strings of questions about symptoms which the patient does not have may well be falsely reassuring to both the doctor and the patient. The entry in the notes, *'Dysuria. No discharge. Given Trimethoprim'* implies that the doctor thought of an STI as a possibility, but dismissed it (on erroneous grounds).

Symptom questions *are* valuable in some circumstances. For example, the severity of pelvic inflammatory disease needs to be carefully assessed to help aid a decision as to whether admission is indicated. Again, in the difficult circumstance when the GP is wondering if HIV disease is a possibility, gathering further evidence by asking about, for example, weight loss, sweats or diarrhoea, can be helpful.

Taking a partner history

Despite its title, the partner history is not used to check if the *partner* has symptoms, but rather aims to clarify the patient's sexual partnerships. A pragmatic approach is to take the history back to the most recent apparent risk (see *How far back should we take the risk assessment,* page 53). Whether the most recent risk was last month or six years ago, the partner history back to that point is often elicited quickly: partner history-taking is usually quite a quick process.

While some useful questions are suggested below, flexibility is clearly essential. The questions you ask will often be informed by what the patient has already said in the consultation, and sometimes by what you know of the patient. But be aware that this is perhaps the easiest part of the sexual history in which to make wrongful assumptions. *'My husband and I thought I should try a change to the coil'* enables you to make some assumptions, but not others.

Here are some suggested partner history questions. Those shown in square brackets can often be omitted because of information already given in the consultation.

['*Do you have a partner at present?*']
['*Is it a sexual relationship?*']
'*How long have you been together?*'
['*Could I just check – is your partner a man or a woman?*']
'*Do you have any other partners?*'
'*Does your partner have any other partners?*'

['*Have you ever had a sexual relationship?*']
['*When was your last sexual relationship?*']

These simple questions are incredibly useful in primary care. '*Does your partner have any other partners?*' can elicit a cheery assertive '*Heavens no – we're married!*', or a rueful '*Well, you never know, do you?*' These patients may well require completely different approaches: consent to test is almost implicit in the latter response, and almost precluded by the former.

Asking about sexual practices – when is it appropriate?

These are among the most intimate questions that a clinician can ask. It is important for both the clinician and patient to have a clear idea of why the questions are clinically appropriate. You may need to ask specific questions about sexual practices:

- When trying to work out the likelihood of transmission of STI, for example, in a same-sex relationship. Helps to identify when other swab sampling sites may be needed.

- To provide the right advice about condom type. There is currently debate as to whether stronger condoms are safer for anal intercourse. Use of lubricant (which should be water-based) may reduce trauma to the condom and so be safer.

- In initial assessment of a possible problem with sexual function. *'In order that I find the right type of advice for you, could I ask in a little more detail what you mean?'* This will help to ascertain what type of sexual dysfunction is being referred to.

Assessing condom use

Questions about condom use are much more important if the partner history has revealed potential risk. In other words, if the patient has described a mutually monogamous ten-year marriage, you might omit an assessment of condom use if the clinical context makes this appropriate (that is, you are not considering an AIDS diagnosis). Careful and consistent condom use can be highly protective from some STIs. The reasons why a couple may fail to use a condom – or use one incorrectly – are many. One question is not enough! Use open approaches:

'Do you use condoms?'
'Are there times you haven't managed to use them?'
'Quite a lot of people have difficulties with condoms – do you?'
'Do you have any questions about their use?'

Assessing current contraceptive use

Questions need to be tailored to the individual method used (and non-user-dependent methods such as contraceptive implants may need a little discussion). (See also Chapter 3.)

'Are you happy with your contraceptive method?'
'Do you sometimes find it hard to remember to take the pill?'
'When was the last time that you missed a pill? What did you do?'
'Can you tell me how you normally take your pills over the course of four weeks? Do you ever vary from that?'
'Have you ever had an unplanned pregnancy?'

Considering a start or change of contraceptive method

'Have you considered what method you would like?'
'How important is it for you not to become pregnant?'

Additional assessment for HIV risk

There are additional risks of HIV infection that may need to be assessed. These risks are:

- use of injected drugs

- overseas *travel* (unprotected sexual intercourse; treatment (for example, transfusions) or intravenous drug use)

- overseas *origin*, most notably from countries with a higher prevalence of HIV (unprotected sexual intercourse; treatment (for example, transfusions) or IV drug use)

- risks of partners (men who have sex with men; IV drug users; overseas origin).

Many individuals in risk groups have already thought about HIV, and may even have had tests. But do not close your mind to the possibility that HIV infection can be present in someone at *no* apparent risk – be guided by the clinical circumstances, and be cautious before dissuading people from having an HIV test.

Future risk

Sometimes you are trying to assess possible *future* risk in order to give advice:

[Travel advice]:
'Are you travelling with a partner?'
'Do you think it possible you may have sex with a new partner while you are there?'
'Were you planning to take condoms with you?'

[Contraception]:
'Starting on the pill will help protect you from getting pregnant, but will not protect you from sexually transmissible infections. Do you plan to continue to use condoms? How long do you think you will continue to use them?'

Other useful questions

'Do you have any questions about sexual health that you would like to ask?'
'Do you have any problems with sex that you would like to discuss?'

These questions give the patient an opportunity to raise any issues that you have not covered.

'Have you ever had a sexually transmissible infection?'

Unlike other health problems, there may be no record in primary care of past STIs.

'Have you ever had sex you didn't want and/or agree to?'

Sexual abuse can lead directly to sexual health problems through infections or unplanned pregnancy. It can also lead to psychological problems. However there is also evidence that it can affect risk-taking behaviours and so affect future risk of sexual health problems. It may be that a current partner is controlling or abusive, and this may affect risk-taking behaviour if the patient does not feel able to negotiate preferred behaviours – for example, condom use or mutual monogamy.

There is limited evidence about the acceptability to patients of routine questions about experience of forced sex. One primary care based study of women attenders compared the views of those who reported experience of sexual violence with those who did not[10]. Although there were significant differences between the groups, in both groups the majority reported that it would be 'alright' to be routinely asked by a clinician whether they had experienced sexual assault. In an individual consultation, the decision by the clinician to ask about forced sex may be far from routine. The clinical context, perhaps coupled with clues from the patient, may prompt the clinician to explore this possibility.

How far back should we take the risk assessment?

This will be influenced by the reason you are taking a partner history in the first place. At one extreme, a possible AIDS diagnosis may be the result of a sexual contact 12 years previously. Chlamydia too can be present for years. For gonorrhoea, it is likely that the time span reduces to weeks. Often a partner history and assessment of condom use is being taken to discover whether there is any risk of STI at all – in this instance, going back to the most recent risk is a sufficient and pragmatic approach, which can be used to demonstrate the need to test. However, it is important to avoid implying *who* might have given *what* to *whom*

Interpreting the risk assessment

Remember that risk assessment can inform clinical judgement, but it is a process of *estimation* rather than an accurate measurement. Interpretation of the sexual history often depends on why the clinician decided to take a sexual history in the first place (see *Why and when to use sexual history-taking*, page 39).

Patients at no apparent risk of STI

These patients are an important group in primary care. They include:

- those who have never had sex
- those in a mutual first sexual relationship.

Recognition of this 'no apparent risk' group is important because it:

- empowers patients
- reinforces messages about how infections are transmitted and the benefits of limiting partner changes.

It is not the clinician's place to disbelieve the patient's partner history, unless the clinical picture is compellingly suggestive of an STI – perhaps classic pelvic inflammatory disease or an AIDS diagnosis. In this case, it is important to draw attention to the difficulty: *'Your history suggests that you cannot be at risk of a sexually transmissible infection. My difficulty is that there is little else that is likely to be causing symptoms such as these. Do you think we should test for sexually transmissible infections anyway? How would you feel if the test was positive?'*

Ensure that responsibility for an assessment of 'no risk' is kept with the patient, by using phrases such as, *'If what you tell me is correct, then of course this couldn't be caused by chlamydia.'* The patient may well mull this over after the consultation, and will sometimes return at a later date, if they decide that perhaps they are at risk after all. But when talking to 'no apparent risk' patients, it must not be forgotten that:

- there may still be a risk of unplanned pregnancy
- there may be *future* possible risk, which may need to be mentioned and/or assessed.

Patients at very slight or no risk

It is not too uncommon to encounter patients for whom there is an extremely remote – perhaps almost academic – risk of having an STI: for example, a woman who has not had sex for nine years and who has developed menorrhagia. Some patients with a remote risk will nevertheless be relaxed about a test for an STI; others may be sceptical or reluctant, for a variety of reasons. In these instances, share the diagnostic options with the patient and allow them to determine what will be prioritised.

No risk since last test can also be important for some infections. Patients (especially those who have had an STI in the past) can become quite concerned that the infection could have come back, or they may disbelieve test results that show no infection is present. The roots to this may be psychological, and it is as well not to do repeated tests if they are not indicated.

No sexual intercourse for a length of time that exceeds the time span of a given infection is also indicative of very slight/no risk. As there may be plenty of other possible causes for a patient's symptoms, it may be more appropriate to focus on these first; the outside chance of an STI can be revisited later, if need be.

Perfect condom use. Just occasionally, a patient is encountered who has taken meticulous control of their sexual health, and has had no genital contact without condoms. The clinician should take this into account when interpreting risk with the patient. If an STI is a possibility, at least acknowledge to the patient that condoms generally offer very good (though not always perfect) protection, if used correctly.

Patients at moderate to high risk

For the purposes of *diagnosis*, explain to the patient why you would like to test for STIs. For the purposes of *health promotion advice*, explain to the patient why you are concerned, and advise how they can best protect their sexual health. You should now be in a good position to tailor advice to the patient's individual circumstances.

Patients who have had more than three partners in the last 12 months can be considered to be at very high risk of STI, especially if they do not use condoms, or use them erratically. They may benefit from careful advice, even if tests reveal they do not yet have infection. It may be worth discussing hepatitis B testing and immunisation.

'So do you think she gave me something, doctor?'

The role of the GP or practice nurse is *not* forensic; it is generally very unwise to imply that you can tell who gave what to whom. The history may only have been taken back to the most recent risk, but it is often possible that the infection was present before any current relationship. The most important thing is to emphasise that most infections are highly treatable, and that it is better to know about them than *not* to know about them.

Future risk and behaviour change

In most consultations on sexual health, consideration will have to be given to the future risk of the patient. At this stage it is likely to be transparent to the patient how to reduce the risk of having an unplanned pregnancy, acquiring an STI or even perhaps developing cervical cancer. The clinician may need to summarise or re-emphasise aspects of behaviour relevant to the individual patient.

Key messages

- Try to break learned patterns which can inappropriately separate different aspects of sexual health.

- Try to keep the process of sexual history-taking transparent: the patient should be aware of why personal questions are being asked and that their answers will contribute to their clinical management.

- Taking a careful sexual history can give useful insights to the patient and forms part of the basis of informed consent for relevant clinical interventions.

- Give patients clear information about the risks associated with unprotected sex.

- Patients at no apparent risk of STI are an important but diverse group in primary care, and they require particular consideration (discussed in the chapter).

References

1. Churchill D. Consultation patterns and provision of contraception in general practice before teenage pregnancy: case-control study. *British Medical Journal*, vol 321, no 7259, 2000, pp486–89.

2. Pimenta J et al. Opportunistic screening for genital chlamydial infection. II: Prevalence among healthcare attenders, outcome and evaluation of positive cases. *Sexually Transmitted Infection*, vol 79, no 1, 2003, pp22–27.

3. Madge S et al. Access to medical care one year prior to diagnosis in 100 HIV-positive women. *Family Practice*, vol 14, no 3, 1997, pp255–57.

4. Jeal N and Salisbury C. Self-reported experiences of health services among female street-based prostitutes: a cross-sectional survey. *British Journal of General Practice*, vol 54, no 504, 2004, 515–19.

5. *CDR Weekly* vol 12, no 48, November 2002.

6. Johnson A et al. Who goes to sexually transmitted disease clinics? Results from a national population survey. *Genitourinary Medicine,* vol 72, no 3, 1996, pp197–202.

7. Fitzpatrick R et al. Perceptions of general practice among homosexual men. *British Journal of General Practice*, vol 44, no 379, 1994, pp80–82.

8. See note 1 above.

9. See notes 1 and 6 above.

10. Coid J et al. Sexual violence against adult women primary care attenders in east London. *British Journal of General Practice*, vol 53, no 496, 2003, pp858–62.

Chapter 3

CONTRACEPTION

Philip Hannaford

INTRODUCTION

This chapter summarises the main issues involved when giving advice about contraception. Several expert groups have provided advice on the medical criteria for different aspects of contraception[1,2,3,4,5]. Those which have been particularly useful in putting together this chapter include: the World Health Organization (WHO) document, *Improving Access to Quality Care in Family Planning: Medical Eligibility Criteria for Contraceptive Use*[6], the *UK Medical Eligibility Criteria for Contraceptive Use*[7], the *UK Selected Practice Recommendations for Contraceptive Use*[8] and the *British National Formulary*[9].

In this chapter it is assumed that all women can use a method of contraception, unless there are specific reasons to think otherwise. The number of conditions that limit the use of a particular contraceptive is usually small. For each contraceptive method, the following has been specified:

Do not use with these conditions: Conditions which represent an unacceptable health risk if the contraceptive method is used (marked with ◙ in Table 3.1, page 103).

Use cautiously with these conditions: Conditions where the theoretical or proven risks usually outweigh the advantages of the method, that is, careful clinical judgment is needed, taking into account the severity of the condition and the availability, practicability and acceptability of an alternative method. Usually the method under consideration would be of last choice, and careful follow-up is required. The primary care team may need specialist advice if a woman has one of these conditions (marked with ∇ in Table 3.1, page 103).

Broadly usable with these conditions: Conditions where the advantages of the method generally outweigh any theoretical or proven risks, that is, such conditions do not restrict the use of a method but would be a consideration in its selection; careful follow-up may also be needed (marked with ☼ in Table 3.1, page 103).

NB. If a condition is not mentioned then women who are affected can safely use all contraceptive methods.

This information is summarised for reversible methods in Table 3.1 (see page 103). For some conditions, caution is only necessary while the problem is being treated (for example, avoidance of combined oral contraceptives (COCs) while a woman has active hepatitis). In other situations, the balance of risks and benefits is different when the condition is known about *before* using a particular contraceptive compared with situations when the condition occurs *during* usage. Some cautions are based on theoretical rather than proven risk. Within a particular method, different devices may have different considerations. For these reasons, it is important to consider the more detailed information in the separate sections on each method.

Personal preferences about individual products, or groups of products, within each contraceptive method have not been given. This is because consensus can be difficult to reach. In addition, choices may change in the light of new information, sometimes very rapidly. The availability of as wide a range of preparations as possible is important for tailoring choices to the particular needs of each user.

Space constraints have made it impossible to give details of every circumstance in which different contraceptives might be used, and to provide advice about every problem that might arise while using a particular method of contraception. Instead advice is given for the most common situations faced by providers of contraceptive services. Other valuable sources of practical advice for providers include the *UK Selected Practice Recommendations for Contraceptive Use*[10], *British National Formulary*[11], *Contraception Today*[12], **fpa** *contraceptive leaflets*[13], *Contraception – Your Questions Answered*[14] and the *Handbook of Family Planning and Reproductive Health Care*[15].

THE CHALLENGE

The primary care team has a central role in the provision of contraceptive services in the UK. The team is frequently well placed to offer good advice as it knows an individual's health record and circumstances. Continuity of care can also be provided. While many practices offer excellent services, others have some way to go before they meet the best standards of care.

A model of good practice for contraceptive services in primary care includes:

- Easy access to services with guaranteed patient confidentiality.
- An unhurried consultation with knowledgeable personnel, conducted in clean surroundings.
- The provision of comprehensive information, tailored to the needs of each individual or couple, so that correct choices are made.
- The provision of a full range of contraceptive methods (even if this means liaising with outside agencies).
- Appropriate assessment before, and monitoring during, use of a particular method in order to minimise any real or perceived adverse effects.
- Supplementary up-to-date written information for future reference about the correct use of the chosen method (for example, the highly recommended UK **fpa** contraceptive leaflets).
- Information about who to contact if problems or concerns arise in the future with the chosen contraceptive.
- Consideration of other aspects of sexual health including the need for: protection against sexually transmissible infections (STIs) (see Chapter 6), addressing psychosexual problems (see Chapter 8), well person screening (see Chapter 9).
- Review of the chosen method to check that it remains the most appropriate choice.
- Full use of the different skills, training and resources of each member of the primary care team, in particular (well-trained) practice nurses.

The challenge is to enable all service users to feel that they have made the appropriate choice for their circumstances, in an informed and unhurried manner. Pressures of everyday general practice, especially those of time, can sometimes undermine efforts to meet this challenge. Nonetheless, many practices are able to show that it can be done. These practices are usually well organised, with appropriate human and material resources.

The provision of regular, dedicated, family planning sessions helps with providing services for: first visits; women with more complex contraceptive problems; and those wishing to use methods, such as diaphragms, implants or intrauterine devices and systems (IUD and IUS), which initially require more time.

Decisions about the choice of contraception involve a number of considerations: the effectiveness, reversibility, perceived safety, recognised contraindications, acceptability, ease of use and availability of each method. Social and cultural factors are also important. Contraceptive choices for family spacing may be different to those for family limitation (having no more children).

Most contraceptive users are likely to use more than one method during their lifetime. Some women, such as those not in a stable long-term relationship, may need to consider using two methods simultaneously, for example, oral contraceptives to prevent pregnancy and a male or female condom to protect against STIs. However, at the end of the day choice is dependent on confidence with both the method selected and with the service provider (the second of which is related directly to the provision and standard of care).

RELATIVE EFFECTIVENESS OF AVAILABLE METHODS

The reliability of each contraceptive method depends on its inherent effectiveness when used under ideal conditions, and the ability of couples to use it correctly and consistently in everyday life[16]. Avoidable pregnancies can also be caused by omissions and errors on the part of service providers. Table 3.2 (page 110) shows the failure rates of different methods and Table 3.3 (page 110) the estimated risk of pregnancy among women at different ages who do not use contraception.

Providers of contraceptive services often need to assess whether it is reasonably certain that a user is not pregnant. One can reasonably assume absence of pregnancy if the woman has no symptoms or signs of pregnancy and either:

- has not had intercourse since the last normal menses
- has been correctly and consistently using a reliable method of contraception
- is within the first seven days after normal menses
- is within four weeks post-partum for non-lactating women
- is within the first seven days post-abortion or miscarriage
- is fully or nearly fully breastfeeding, amenorrhoeic, and less than six months post-partum[17].

Progestogen-only contraceptive injections

Description

Long acting progestogens given by deep intramuscular injection: Depot medroxyprogesterone acetate (DMPA; Depo-Provera) is given every 12 weeks; norethisterone enanthate (NET-EN: Noristerat) is licensed to be repeated once only after eight weeks. Main effects: inhibition of ovulation; changes in cervical mucus making it hostile to sperm penetration; and endometrial changes.

Advantages

- Highly effective, non-intercourse related contraceptive.
- Can often be used by women with conditions which preclude the use of COCs.
- Does not interfere with breastfeeding.
- May be particularly advantageous in women with a history of venous thrombosis, endometriosis or sickle cell disease.
- May reduce risk of endometrial cancer (DMPA) and may offer some protection against pelvic inflammatory disease.
- The reliable prevention of ovulation provides protection against ectopic pregnancy and functional ovarian cysts.
- Can be used as an alternative to COCs before major surgery, before all surgery to the legs, or before surgery that involves prolonged immobilisation of a lower limb.

Disadvantages

- Once given, any side effects are irreversible for the remaining duration of action (that is, up to two to three months).
- Temporary delay in return of regular periods and fertility (DMPA: median fertility delay nine months after last injection).
- Irregular bleeding, including excessive and more frequent.
- Amenorrhoea (DMPA rather than Noristerat).
- Weight gain (DMPA rather than Noristerat).
- Severe headaches may increase in frequency.
- Progestogen-only contraceptives and possible associations with breast cancer have not been extensively researched, but the limited data available suggests

a similar pattern of risk of breast cancer as that found for combined oral contraceptives[18].

- Does not protect against STIs.

Do not use with these conditions (◉)
- Pregnancy.
- Current breast cancer.

Use cautiously with these conditions (▽)
- Gestational trophoblastic neoplasia, while hCG levels are abnormal (no restriction once levels become normal).
- Multiple risk factors for arterial cardiovascular disease (such as older age, smoking, diabetes and hypertension).
- Hypertension, controlled with vascular disease.
- Current deep vein thrombosis (DVT) or pulmonary embolism (PE) (theoretically progestogen-only contraceptives may increase the risk of thrombosis although the risk is probably substantially less than for COCs).
- Ischaemic heart disease.
- Stroke.
- Migraine with aura, *if onset occurs during use*.
- Diabetes *with* nephropathy/retinopathy/neuropathy/other vascular disease, or duration more than 20 years.
- Breast cancer: past history with no evidence of current disease for at least five years.
- Unexplained vaginal bleeding (important to exclude serious underlying illness, especially before initiating use of an injection).
- Active viral hepatitis.
- Severe (decompensated) liver cirrhosis.
- Liver tumours (benign or malignant).

Broadly usable with these conditions (☼)
- Before age 18 if no other contraceptive method is suitable. This relates to concerns about possible effects on bone mineral density[19].
- After age 45 (theoretical concerns about hypo-estrogenic effects (especially of DMPA) and whether bone mass loss is regained after discontinuation).

- Questionable fertility from whatever reason.
- Breastfeeding less than six weeks post-partum (theoretical concern about effects of neonatal exposure to steroids during this period; bleeding irregularities more common).
- Controlled hypertension without vascular disease.
- Blood pressure consistently elevated, systolic ≥ 160 or diastolic ≥ 95 mm Hg.
- History of DVT /PE.
- Known thrombogenic mutations (for example, Factor V Leiden, Prothrombin mutation, Protein S, Protein C and Antithrombin deficiencies).
- Major surgery with prolonged immobilisation.
- Known hyperlipidaemia.
- Migraine: current problem without aura; current problem with aura, *if onset occurred before use*; or past problem with aura.
- Diabetes without vascular disease.
- Breast disease: undiagnosed mass.
- Breast cancer: carrier of gene mutations known to be associated with elevated risk (for example, BRCA 1).
- Abnormal vaginal bleeding patterns: irregular without heavy bleeding, or with heavy or prolonged bleeding (including regular or irregular patterns).
- Cervical intraepithelial neoplasia (CIN) awaiting treatment.
- Cervical cancer awaiting treatment.
- Acquired immune deficiency syndrome (AIDS) and using highly active anti-retroviral therapy (HAART).
- Gallbladder/biliary tract disease, including asymptomatic disease.
- History of COC-related cholestasis.
- Mild (compensated) liver cirrhosis.
- Raynaud's disease: secondary with lupus anticoagulant.
- Antiretroviral therapy (consult local human immunodeficiency virus (HIV) specialist or refer to www.hiv-druginteractions.org).

Initial assessment before injection

The prolonged action of injectable contraceptives means that they should not be used without full counselling, backed up by a patient information leaflet. A careful personal and family medical history with particular attention to cardiovascular risk factors, and an accurate blood pressure measurement is sufficient for most women. Further assessment is needed only if a relevant personal or family history is disclosed, or if blood pressure is elevated. Enquiries should also be made about future pregnancy intentions, especially whether the user wishes to get pregnant immediately after the injection becomes ineffective (DMPA is associated with a temporary delay in return to fertility). There is no need for routine screening by means of physical examination (including breast and bimanual pelvic examination), urine or blood test, before using a contraceptive injection. Indeed, the routine use of such procedures can restrict accessibility to use of an injection, as well as other methods of contraception.

Give first injection within first five days of the menstrual cycle to avoid the need for extra contraception (otherwise use additional contraception for seven days). Post-partum: give between 21–28 days after delivery (delaying to six weeks if fully breastfeeding) to avoid the need for extra contraception (otherwise use additional contraception for seven days). Use after abortion or miscarriage: can be provided immediately if pregnancy less than 24 weeks. After this time treat as if normal pregnancy.

Monitoring during usage

The follow-up assessment should include enquiries about any problems, especially the development of new or more severe headaches and an assessment of any abnormal bleeding patterns. Many practitioners check the user's blood pressure before every injection although there is little evidence on which to base this practice. Little is known about the effects of contraceptive injections on blood pressure.

Repeat injections can be given up to two weeks late without the need for additional contraception. If given more than two weeks late, use additional contraception for seven days. Switching between DMPA and NET-EN is not recommended. If a switch is necessary, change when the repeat injection is due.

Progestogen-only contraceptive implants

Description

Single flexible rod inserted subdermally into the upper arm, releasing small amounts of etonorgestrel (Implanon); effective for three years. Norplant (six polydimethylsiloxane implants of levonorgestrel which lasts for five years) is no longer available in the UK but some women may still have the rods in situ. Main effects: inhibition of ovulation; changes in cervical mucus making it hostile to sperm penetration; endometrial changes.

Advantages

- Highly effective, non-intercourse related contraceptive.
- Effects rapidly reversed after removal.
- Can often be used by women with conditions which preclude the use of COCs.
- Biological effects less than progestogen-only injections; more like progestogen-only pill (POP).
- Does not interfere with breastfeeding.
- Can be used as an alternative to COCs before major surgery, before all surgery to the legs, or before surgery that involves prolonged immobilisation of a lower limb.

Disadvantages

- Once given, any side effects are irreversible until the rod is removed.
- Irregular bleeding, including excessive, prolonged, more frequent or absent, especially in the first few months.
- Insertion requires small surgical procedure under local anaesthetic: *potential risk of infection, bruising and itch at insertion site; migration of the rod; difficulties with removal.*
- Reported side effects include acne, nausea, headaches, hair loss or growth and weight gain.
- Does not protect against STIs.

Do not use with these conditions (◉)

- Pregnancy.
- Current breast cancer.

Use cautiously with these conditions (▽)

- Gestational trophoblastic neoplasia, while hCG levels are abnormal (no restriction once levels become normal).
- Current DVT/PE.
- Ischaemic heart disease, *if diagnosis occurs during use*.
- Stroke, *if occurs during use*.

- Migraine with aura, *if onset occurs during use*.
- Breast cancer: past history with no evidence of current disease for at least five years.
- Unexplained vaginal bleeding (important to exclude serious underlying illness, especially before insertion).
- Active viral hepatitis.
- Severe (decompensated) liver cirrhosis.
- Liver tumours (benign or malignant).
- Use of drugs which induce liver enzymes (for example, barbiturates, carbamazepine, griseofulvin, modafinil, oxcarbazepine, phenytoin, primidone, rifabutin, rifampicin, topiramate and some complementary medicines such as St John's wort).

Broadly usable with these conditions (☼)

- Questionable fertility from whatever reason.
- Multiple risk factors for arterial cardiovascular disease (such as older age, smoking, diabetes and hypertension).
- Controlled hypertension with vascular disease.
- History of DVT/PE.
- Known thrombogenic mutations (for example, Factor V Leiden, Prothrombin mutation, Protein S, Protein C and Antithrombin deficiencies).
- Major surgery with prolonged immobilisation.
- Ischaemic heart disease, *if diagnosis occurred before insertion*.
- Stroke, *if occurred before insertion*.
- Known hyperlipidaemia.
- Migraine: current problem without aura; current problem with aura, *if onset occurred before use*; or past problem with aura.
- Diabetes with or without vascular disease.
- Breast disease: undiagnosed mass.
- Breast cancer: carrier of gene mutations known to be associated with elevated risk (for example, BRCA 1).
- Abnormal vaginal bleeding patterns: irregular without heavy bleeding, or with heavy or prolonged bleeding (including regular or irregular patterns).

- Cervical cancer awaiting treatment.

- HIV positive, *if receiving anti-retroviral therapy*.

- AIDS and using HAART.

- Gallbladder/biliary tract disease, including asymptomatic disease.

- History of COC-related cholestasis.

- Mild (compensated) liver cirrhosis.

- Raynaud's disease: secondary with lupus anticoagulant.

- Antiretroviral therapy (consult local HIV specialist or refer to www.hiv-druginteractions.org).

Initial assessment before insertion

The prolonged action of contraceptive implants means that they should not be used without full counselling, backed up by a patient information leaflet. A careful personal and family medical history with particular attention to cardiovascular risk factors, and an accurate blood pressure measurement is sufficient for most women. Further assessment is needed only if a relevant personal or family history is disclosed, or if blood pressure is elevated. Routine screening by means of physical examination (including breast and bimanual pelvic examination), urine or blood tests should not be a prerequisite before inserting an implant. Indeed, the routine use of such procedures can restrict accessibility to use of an implant, as well as other methods of contraception.

Implants should only be inserted and removed by providers who have been adequately trained. Progestogen-only implants should be inserted within the first five days of the menstrual cycle to avoid the need for extra contraception (otherwise use additional contraception for seven days). Post-partum: insert between days 21–28 after delivery to avoid the need for extra contraception. Use after abortion or miscarriage: can be inserted immediately if pregnancy is less than 24 weeks. After this time treat as if normal pregnancy.

Monitoring during usage

The follow-up assessment should enquire about any problems, especially the development of new or more severe headaches, and any abnormal bleeding patterns.

Concomitant use of other drugs

Short-term use of a liver enzyme-inducing drug requires additional contraception while taking the enzyme-inducing drug and until four weeks after stopping it. Rifampicin and rifabutin are such powerful liver enzyme-inducing drugs that even if the course lasts for less than seven days (for example, a two day course to eliminate carriage of meningococcus), extra contraception is needed until four weeks after stopping. Women taking liver enzyme-inducing drugs long term, *especially rifampicin or rifabutin,* should consider another method of contraception, such as an IUD.

Levonorgestrel-releasing intrauterine system (IUS)

Description

T shaped plastic device which releases a small daily dose of levonorgestrel (about a third of that of a POP) from its polydimethylsiloxane reservoir through a rate-limiting membrane for at least five years. Main effects are local: endometrial suppression, changes to cervical mucus and uterotubal fluid; suppression of ovulation in some women, in some cycles.

Advantages

Contraceptive

- Highly effective, non-intercourse related contraceptive.
- Rapid return of fertility after removal.
- Can often be used by women with conditions which preclude the use of COCs.
- Immediately effective.
- Does not interfere with breastfeeding.

Non-contraceptive

- Reduced blood loss, sometimes amenorrhoea (after several months' usage), modest rises in haemoglobin levels (may make this the contraceptive of choice for women with very heavy menses).
- Less dysmenorrhoea.
- Possibly reduced risk of clinical pelvic inflammatory disease (PID).
- Possibly reduced risk of extra-uterine pregnancies (because of its great efficiency at reducing all pregnancies whatever their site).

Disadvantages

- Expulsion (risk of pregnancy).

- Uterine or cervical perforation (highly dependent on the service provider, can result in risk of pregnancy; risk of bowel/bladder adhesions).

- Infection (greatest risk in first 20 days after insertion, probably related to pre-existing carriage of infection, before reverting to background risk of STIs).

- Hormonal side effects in first few months after insertion, including irregular usually light, uterine bleeding, increased duration of vaginal bleeding and functional ovarian cysts.

- No research is available to show it is effective as an emergency contraceptive, and therefore it cannot be recommended for this purpose especially since it may be slightly slower to take effect than the copper IUD.

- Does not protect against STIs.

Do not use with these conditions (◉)

- Pregnancy.

- Puerperal sepsis.

- Immediately after septic abortion.

- Gestational trophoblastic neoplasia, while hCG levels are abnormal (no restriction once levels become normal).

- Current breast cancer.

- Unexplained vaginal bleeding (important to exclude serious underlying illness), *if present before insertion*.

- Cervical cancer awaiting treatment, *if diagnosis occurred before use*.

- Endometrial cancer, *if diagnosis occurred before use*.

- Uterine fibroids distorting uterine cavity.

- Severely distorted uterine cavity, cavity less than 5.5mm.

- PID – current (or within last three months) at time of intended insertion.

- STI, including purulent cervicitis, chlamydial infection or gonorrhoea – current (or within last three months) at time of intended insertion.

- Pelvic tuberculosis, *if known about at time of intended insertion*.

- Strong immunosuppression (but standard regimens of corticosteroids are not a risk).

Use cautiously with these conditions (∇)

- Less than four weeks post-partum (because of: concerns about perforation especially if breastfeeding; effects on uterine involution) *NB*. More usual time of insertion is about six to eight weeks post-partum. Insertion can occur from four weeks post-partum.

- Current DVT/PE.

- Ischaemic heart disease, *if diagnosis occurs during use*.

- Migraine with aura, *if onset occurs during use*.

- Breast cancer: past history with no evidence of current disease for at least five years.

- Ovarian cancer, *if diagnosis occurred before use*.

- Increased risk of STIs, *if present before use*.

- Pelvic tuberculosis, *if diagnosis made during use*.

- Active viral hepatitis.

- Severe (decompensated) liver cirrhosis.

- Liver tumours: benign or malignant.

- Antiretroviral therapy, *if need is present before use* (consult local HIV specialist or refer to www.hiv-druginteractions.org).

Broadly usable with these conditions (☼)

- Age less than 20 (concerns about risk of expulsion because of nulliparity).

- Questionable fertility for whatever reason.

- Multiple risk factors for arterial cardiovascular disease (such as older age, smoking, diabetes and hypertension).

- Controlled hypertension with vascular disease.

- History of DVT/PE.

- Known thrombogenic mutations (for example, Factor V Leiden, Prothrombin mutation, Protein S, Protein C and Antithrombin deficiencies).

- Major surgery with prolonged immobilisation.

- Ischaemic heart disease, *if diagnosis occurred before use*.

- Structural valvular or congenital heart disease, *if complicated* (for example, by pulmonary hypertension, atrial fibrillation or history of subacute bacterial endocarditis) [NB. needs antibiotic cover at insertion].

- Stroke.

- Known hyperlipidaemia.

- Migraine: current problem without aura; current problem with aura, *if onset occurred before use*; or past problem with aura.

- Diabetes with or without vascular disease.

- Breast disease: undiagnosed mass.

- Breast cancer: carrier of gene mutations known to be associated with elevated risk (for example, BRCA 1).

- Unexplained vaginal bleeding (important to exclude serious underlying illness), *if occurs during use*.

- Heavy or prolonged vaginal bleeding (including regular patterns), *if occurs during use*.

- CIN awaiting treatment.

- Cervical cancer awaiting treatment, *if diagnosis occurs during use*.

- Ovarian cancer, *if diagnosis occurs during use*.

- Endometrial cancer, *if diagnosis occurs during use*.

- Anatomic abnormalities interfering with insertion, for example, cervical stenosis.

- Past history of PID (assuming no known current risk factors for STIs) without subsequent pregnancy.

- PID, *if onset occurs during use*.

- STI, including purulent cervicitis, chlamydial infection, gonorrhoea, other STIs and vaginitis, *if onset occurs during use*.

- Increased risk of STIs, *if develops during use*.

- HIV positive, irrespective of whether receiving anti-retroviral therapy.

- AIDS and using HAART.

- Increased risk of HIV/AIDS.

- Gallbladder/biliary tract disease, including asymptomatic disease.

- Past COC-related cholestasis.

- Mild (compensated) liver cirrhosis.

- Raynaud's disease: secondary with lupus anticoagulant.

- Antiretroviral therapy, *if the need occurs during use* (consult local HIV specialist or refer to www.hiv-druginteractions.org).

NB. Many of the concerns mentioned above reflect the current lack of information about the effects of the progestogen provided by the system. The daily dosage, however, is less than the daily dose of POP. Many concerns, therefore, are theoretical rather than proven. Indeed the system may be particularly useful for some women with some of the above conditions if alternative contraceptives are unsatisfactory. Liver enzyme-inducing drugs are unlikely to significantly reduce the contraceptive efficacy of the IUS.

Initial assessment before insertion

Before insertion, careful counselling should be given, backed up by a patient information leaflet. A careful personal medical history with particular attention to gynaecological history and risk factors for STIs is required. Ideally all women should be screened for STIs, particularly Chlamydia trachomatis, before insertion. Prophylactic antibiotics are not generally recommended for IUS insertion, although they may be useful in areas with both high prevalence of STIs and limited screening facilities. Blind treatment with broad-spectrum antibiotics, however, is a second best option as the opportunity for contact tracing is lost, thereby increasing the risk of reinfection.

IUSs should only be inserted by providers who have been adequately trained. Insert within first seven days of the menstrual cycle (anytime if replacement) to avoid the need for extra contraception (otherwise use additional contraception for seven days). The IUS can be inserted immediately after an abortion or miscarriage if the pregnancy is less than 24 weeks. After this time treat as a normal pregnancy. Users should be advised to attend, *as an emergency,* if they develop persistent pain during the first 20 days after insertion.

Monitoring during usage

Menstrual patterns are often changed in the first months of use (for example, spotting or prolonged bleeding). The follow-up assessment should enquire about any problems, especially pain and bleeding. Either symptom should be assumed to be due to one of the complications (infection, ectopic pregnancy, miscarriage, malposition), and excluded from the differential diagnosis before attributing them as side effects of the IUS. Assessment (after first menses or three to six weeks after insertion, then perhaps annually) should check for side effects and other problems, with possible examination for partial expulsion/malposition and pelvic tenderness.

Copper-bearing intrauterine devices (IUDs)

Description

Intrauterine device of copper wire curved round different shaped pieces of plastic or crimped to a polypropylene thread (GyneFix). Main effects: prevents fertilisation; blocks endometrial implantation.

Advantages

- Highly effective, non-intercourse related contraceptive.
- Effects reverse rapidly after removal.
- Can often be used by women with conditions which preclude the use of COCs, such as a history of venous thrombosis.
- Fertility declines with age, so a copper IUD in a woman over 40 can provide continuous contraception until the menopause.
- Immediately effective.
- Useful for emergency contraception (see later).
- Does not interfere with breastfeeding.

Disadvantages

- Intrauterine pregnancy (miscarriage risk).
- Extrauterine pregnancy (although the absolute risk of pregnancy is reduced, the fewer pregnancies which occur are more likely to be ectopic).
- Expulsion (risk of pregnancy).
- Uterine or cervical perforation (highly dependent on the service provider, can result in risk of pregnancy; risk of bowel/bladder adhesions).
- Infection (greatest risk in first 20 days after insertion, probably related to pre-existing carriage of infection, before reverting to background risk of STI).
- Pain (except GyneFix).
- Vaginal bleeding (increased amount/duration).
- Does not protect against STIs.

Do not use with these conditions (◉)

- Pregnancy.
- Puerperal sepsis.
- Immediately after septic abortion.

- Gestational trophoblastic neoplasia, while hCG levels are abnormal (no restriction once levels become normal).
- Unexplained vaginal bleeding (important to exclude serious underlying illness), *if present before insertion*.
- Cervical cancer awaiting treatment, *if diagnosis occurred before use*.
- Endometrial cancer, *if diagnosis occurred before use*.
- Uterine fibroid distorting uterine cavity.
- Severely distorted uterine cavity, cavity less than 5.5mm.
- PID – current (or within last 3 months) at time of intended insertion.
- STI, including purulent cervicitis, chlamydial infection or gonorrhoea – current (or within last 3 months) at time of intended insertion.
- Pelvic tuberculosis, *if diagnosis made during use*.
- Wilson's disease.
- Allergy to copper.
- Strong immunosuppression (but standard regimens of corticosteroids are not a risk).

Use cautiously with these conditions (∇)

- Less than four weeks post-partum (because of concerns about perforation especially if breastfeeding) *NB*. More usual time of insertion is about six to eight weeks post-partum. Insertion can occur from four weeks post-partum.
- Current DVT/PE (because of possibility of increased bleeding in association with anticoagulation therapy).
- Ovarian cancer, *if diagnosis occurred before use*.
- Increased risk of STIs, *if present before use*.
- Pelvic tuberculosis, *if diagnosis made during use*.
- Antiretroviral therapy, *if need is present before use* (consult local HIV specialist or refer to www.hiv-druginteractions.org).

Broadly usable with these conditions (☼)

- Age less than 20 (concerns about risk of expulsion because of nulliparity).
- Questionable fertility for whatever reason.

- Structural valvular or congenital heart disease, if complicated (for example, by pulmonary hypertension, atrial fibrillation or history of subacute bacterial endocarditis) [NB. needs antibiotic cover at insertion].

- Unexplained vaginal bleeding (important to exclude serious underlying illness), *if occurs during use*.

- Heavy or prolonged vaginal bleeding (including regular patterns).

- Severe dysmenorrhoea.

- Cervical cancer awaiting treatment, *if diagnosis occurs during use*.

- Ovarian cancer, *if diagnosis occurs during use*.

- Endometrial cancer, *if diagnosis occurs during use*.

- Anatomical abnormalities interfering with IUD insertion, such as cervical stenosis.

- Endometriosis.

- Past history of PID (assuming no known current risk factors for STIs) without subsequent pregnancy.

- PID, *if diagnosis occurs during use*.

- STI, including purulent cervicitis, chlamydial infection, gonorrhoea, other STIs and vaginitis, *if present during use*.

- Increased risk of STIs, *if develops during use*.

- HIV positive, irrespective of whether receiving anti-retroviral therapy.

- AIDS and using HAART.

- Increased risk of HIV/AIDS.

- Any severe anaemia: for example, thalassaemia, sickle cell disease, iron deficiency anaemia.

- Antiretroviral therapy, *if the need occurs during use* (consult local HIV specialist or refer to www.hiv-druginteractions.org).

Initial assessment before insertion

A careful personal medical history with particular attention to gynaecological history and risk factors for STIs is required. Ideally all women should be screened for STIs, particularly Chlamydia trachomatis, before insertion. Prophylactic antibiotics are not generally recommended for IUD insertion, although they may be useful in areas with both high prevalence of STIs and limited screening facilities. Blind treatment with broad-spectrum antibiotics, however, is a second best option as the opportunity for contact tracing is lost, thereby increasing the risk of reinfection.

IUDs should only be inserted by providers who have been adequately trained. IUDs can be inserted at any convenient time during the menstrual cycle, provided that it is reasonably certain that the woman is not pregnant; additional contraception is not needed. The IUD can be inserted immediately after an abortion or miscarriage if the pregnancy is less than 24 weeks. After this time treat as a normal pregnancy. Users should be advised to attend, *as an emergency,* if they develop persistent pain during the first 20 days after insertion.

Monitoring during usage

The follow-up assessment should enquire about any problems, especially pain and bleeding. Either symptom should be assumed to be due to one of the complications (infection, ectopic pregnancy, miscarriage, malposition), and excluded from the differential diagnosis before attributing them as side effects of the IUD. Assessment (after first menses or three to six weeks after insertion, then perhaps annually) should check for side effects and other problems, with possible examination for partial expulsion/malposition and pelvic tenderness.

An IUD should not be removed mid-cycle unless additional contraception has been used for the previous seven days. If this has not occurred, and removal is essential, consider emergency contraception. If PID is diagnosed during use, treat the infection with appropriate antibiotics. There is no need to remove the device if the user wishes to continue using it. If not, remove the device *after* antibiotics have been started and consider whether emergency contraception is needed. If an IUD fails, exclude ectopic pregnancy. If the user wishes to continue with the pregnancy, remove the device in the first trimester if possible (reduces the increased risk of second trimester miscarriage, pre-term delivery and infection from a device left in situ, although removal itself carries a small risk of miscarriage). If the device remains in situ, warn the user to return *promptly* if she develops heavy bleeding, cramping, pain, abnormal vaginal discharge or fever.

Combined oral contraceptives (COCs)

Description

Combination of estrogen and progestogen. Main effects: prevention of ovulation; changes to cervical mucus making it hostile to sperm penetration; thinning of endometrium to prevent implantation.

Advantages

Contraceptive

- Highly effective, non-intercourse related, reversible.

Non-contraceptive

- Reduced risk of ovarian and endometrial cancer, protection which increases with duration of use and persists for many years after cessation of COC use.

- Reduction of most disorders of menstruation.

- Users less likely to develop iron deficiency anaemia.

- Fewer functional ovarian cysts.

- Fewer extrauterine pregnancies because normal ovulation inhibited.

- Reduced risk of PID.

- Reduced risk of benign breast disease.

- Probable reduction in rate of endometriosis.

- Fewer symptomatic fibroids.

- Probable reduction in thyroid disease (both overactive and underactive syndromes).

- Possible reduction in risk of rheumatoid arthritis.

- Fewer sebaceous disorders (with estrogen-dominant COCs).

- Possibly fewer duodenal ulcers (not well established and perhaps due to avoidance of COCs by women who are prone to anxiety).

- Reduction in Trichomonas vaginalis infections.

- Possible lower incidence of toxic-shock syndrome.

NB. Most of the evidence for the non-contraceptive benefits comes from studies of women using COCs with higher doses of hormones than currently used. Some of the benefits, therefore, may be smaller with currently available products, although limited evidence suggests that the benefits may be maintained.

Disadvantages

- Requires consistent regular use.

- Increased risk of venous thromboembolic disease in current users, which appears to be highest in the first year of use, and which disappears rapidly after COCs are stopped.

- Increased risk of arterial disease (myocardial infarction, stroke, peripheral vascular disease); mainly (if not entirely) in COC users with other arterial risk factors (for example, smokers, those with raised blood pressure, diabetics, older users). The increased risk in current users disappears when COCs are stopped and is unrelated to duration of use.

- Increases in blood pressure can occur, which usually reverse when COCs are stopped.

- Increase in risk of localised breast cancer being diagnosed while using COCs and for up to ten years after stopping, but *less clinically advanced* disease[20] (the relative risk is unaffected by a family history of breast cancer or personal history of benign breast disease, although both factors increase the background risk of breast cancer so the absolute/ attributable risk is increased).

- Possible increase in risk of cervical cancer in long-term users.

- Possible increase in risk of liver tumours, mainly in long-term users (very rare in British women).

- Possible increased risk of choriocarcinoma in women given COCs in the presence of active trophoblastic disease (hence advice in the UK to avoid using COCs while urine and serum hCG levels are elevated).

- Often associated with a long list of non-bleeding, so-called 'minor' side effects, such as nausea, bloatedness, breast tenderness, tiredness, acne, depression, many of which have not been substantiated by good clinical trial data. Weight has been assessed in a randomised clinical trial, and weight gain or loss was not found to be related to COC use.

- Does not protect against STIs.

NB. The annual incidence of serious disease is very low at the age when most women use COCs (below 35 years). Thus, the absolute number of COC users affected each year is very small. For some conditions (notably arterial disease), this very low risk can be reduced further by a careful assessment before prescribing COCs.

Do not use with these conditions (◉)

- Pregnancy.

- Age 35+ years *and* multiple risk factors for arterial disease (for example, hypertension or diabetes), especially if severe.

- Smoker and aged ≥ 35 years, especially if smokes ≥ 15 cigarettes daily or smokes less then this but has other risk factors for cardiovascular disease.

- Obesity: body mass index (BMI) $\geq$ 40 kg/m^2.

- Breastfeeding (fully or almost fully), less than six weeks post-partum.

- Gestational trophoblastic neoplasia, while hCG levels are abnormal (no restriction once levels become normal).

- Hypertension: controlled with vascular disease.

- Blood pressure consistently elevated, systolic $\geq$ 160 or diastolic $\geq$ 95 mm Hg.

- Current or past DVT/PE.

- Known thrombogenic mutations (for example, Factor V Leiden, Prothrombin mutation, Protein S, Protein C and Antithrombin deficiencies).

- Major surgery with prolonged immobilisation; surgery to legs; prolonged immobilisation after fractures (temporary risk).

- Ischaemic heart disease.

- Structural valvular or congenital heart disease, *if complicated* (for example, by pulmonary hypertension, atrial fibrillation or history of subacute bacterial endocarditis).

- Stroke.

- Migraine: current problem with aura at any age, especially if severe and recurrent (more than once a month); or current problem without aura, *if onset occurs during use among older (age $\geq$ 35) users*.

- Diabetes with vascular disease or more than 20 years duration, *if associated with other arterial risk factors*.

- Current breast cancer.

- Active hepatitis (until liver function returns to normal).

- Severe (decompensated) liver cirrhosis.

- Liver tumours: benign or malignant.

- Raynaud's disease: secondary with lupus anticoagulant.

Use cautiously with these conditions (∇)

- Age 35+ years *and* one risk factor for arterial disease of mild/moderate severity (for example, smoker < 15 cigarettes daily or stopped within previous year, controlled hypertension or uncomplicated diabetes).

- Smoker aged < 35 with multiple risk factors for arterial disease, especially if severe.

- Obesity: body mass index (BMI) 35 to 39 kg/m^2.
- Breastfeeding (fully or almost fully), six weeks to six months post-partum.
- Hypertension: controlled without vascular problems.
- Blood pressure consistently elevated, systolic 140–159 or diastolic 90–94 mm Hg.
- Long term immobilisation (for example, in a wheelchair: avoid use if confined to bed or leg in plaster cast).
- Family history of DVT/PE in a first degree relative aged < 45 years when they had the event.
- Known hyperlipidaemia, especially if severe or with other risk factors for arterial disease.
- Migraine: current problem without aura, especially if severe and recurrent (more than once a month), *if onset occurs before use in older (age 35+) users or during use in younger users*; or past history of migraine with aura at any age.
- Diabetes with vascular disease or more than 20 years duration, *with no other arterial risk factors*.
- Breast disease: undiagnosed mass, *if occurs before use*.
- Breast cancer: past history with no evidence of current disease for at least five years; carrier of gene mutations known to be associated with elevated risk (for example, BRCA 1).
- Gallbladder/biliary tract disease: symptomatic, including disease being medically treated.
- Past history of COC-related cholestasis.
- Mild (compensated) liver cirrhosis.
- Use of drugs which induce liver enzymes (for example, barbiturates, carbamazepine, griseofulvin, modafinil, oxcarbazepine, phenytoin, primidone, rifabutin, rifampicin, topiramate and some complementary medicines such as St John's wort).

Broadly usable with these conditions (☼)
- Aged more than 35 years, if other risk factors for arterial disease (especially smoking) are absent.
- Aged less than 35 years *and* a smoker (regular encouragement to stop smoking, rather than stop COC use is needed).

- Obesity: body mass index (BMI) 30 to 34 kg/m².
- Breastfeeding (medium to low partial), six weeks to six months post-partum.
- History of high blood pressure during pregnancy (where current blood pressure is measurable and normal).
- Major surgery without prolonged immobilisation (temporary risk).
- Family history of DVT/PE in a first degree relative aged ≥ 45 years when they had the event.
- Superficial thrombophlebitis.
- Varicose veins (avoid during sclerosing therapy or if definite history of DVT).
- Structural valvular or congenital heart disease, *if uncomplicated*.
- Known hyperlipidaemia, if mild and no other risk factors for arterial disease.
- Recurrent headaches, including migraine without aura (these become an unacceptable risk if more than once a month and are associated with other significant arterial risk factors (including age over 35), or occur for the first time during use).
- Diabetes without vascular disease.
- Breast disease: undiagnosed mass, *if occurs during use*.
- Unexplained vaginal bleeding (important to exclude serious abnormalities especially before initiating COC use).
- CIN awaiting treatment.
- Cervical cancer awaiting treatment.
- HIV positive, *if receiving anti-retroviral therapy*.
- AIDS and using HAART.
- Gallbladder/biliary tract disease: previously symptomatic treated by cholecystectomy and asymptomatic disease.
- History of pregnancy-related cholestasis.
- Inflammatory bowel disease (includes ulcerative colitis and Crohn's disease).
- Sickle cell disease (but *not* sickle cell trait which is not a problem).
- Raynaud's disease: secondary without lupus anticoagulant.
- Use of antibiotics that do not induce liver enzymes.
- Antiretroviral therapy (consult local HIV specialist or refer to www.hiv-druginteractions.com).

Initial assessment before COC use

Most of the conditions above are rare in young women. A careful personal and family medical history with particular attention to cardiovascular risk factors, and an accurate blood pressure measurement is sufficient for most women[21]. Further assessment is needed only if a relevant personal or family history is disclosed, or the blood pressure is elevated. In general, COCs are broadly usable when there is one risk factor for venous thrombosis (for example, family history, obesity, long-term immobilisation, varicose veins) or arterial disease (for example, family history, diabetes, hypertension, smoking, age over 35, obesity, migraine). If there are two or more risk factors, use more cautiously or avoid use (depending on severity of the combining factors). Routine screening by means of physical examination (including breast and bimanual pelvic examination), urine or blood tests should not be a prerequisite for obtaining COCs. Indeed, the routine use of such procedures can restrict accessibility to use of COCs, as well as other methods of contraception.

Starting the COC

The first visit covers a lot of ground and it is important to make sure that the following is given:

- Up-to-date written information about COCs, with specific details of issues relating to everyday (ED) pills if prescribed.

- Advice that each new pack of pills should be started on the same day of the week.

- Information that even if bleeding occurs while taking the pill, the pack should be finished.

- Advice that intercourse during the pill-free interval is only safe if the next pack is used on time; otherwise alternative contraceptives are required from the last pill in the pack.

- Information that even if bleeding has not stopped, the next pack should be started on time.

- Written advice about: what to do with missed pills; if vomiting occurs; if taking drugs/medicines which interfere with COCs.

- When to seek advice immediately.

- Who is available in the practice to give advice.

Ideally, COCs should be started on day one of the menstrual cycle, but they can be started up to and including day five without the need for additional contraception (otherwise additional contraception is needed for seven days). A woman can switch from one COC brand to another containing a different progestogen immediately without extra contraception, *provided that* she has been using the previous brand consistently and correctly, and it is reasonably certain that she is not pregnant. If changing from a contraceptive injection: start COCs when the next injection is due (no additional contraception is needed).

Monitoring during usage

The follow-up assessment should:

- Enquire about any new risk factors which might have developed.
- Ask about any symptoms, especially headaches.
- Check that the pills are being taken correctly.
- Check the blood pressure.

There is no consensus about how frequently follow-up visits should be. The Faculty of Family Planning and Reproductive Health Care has stated that up to 12 months supply of COC can be given at first and subsequent visits[22]. Many practitioners, however, would arrange an initial follow-up visit after one to three months of starting, to enquire about side effects, discuss any problems and to check the user's blood pressure. Subsequent visits are then six monthly, with perhaps an extension of the interval to annual checks if no problems emerge and the blood pressure remains low after two or three years of use. There is no need for other screening procedures simply because a woman is using COCs.

Missed COCs[23]

If at any time in cycle, **one or two** pills are missed containing 30–35μg ethinylestradiol, or **one** pill is missed containing 20μg ethinylestradiol:

- Take most recent missed pill as soon as it is remembered.
- Discard any earlier missed pills.
- Take the remaining pills in the pack daily at the usual time (may mean taking two pills on the same day – one on remembering and one at the usual time; sometimes this may be the same time).
- No extra contraceptive protection needed.
- No emergency contraception needed.

If at any time in the cycle, **three or more** pills are missed containing 30–35μg ethinylestradiol, or **two or more** pills are missed containing 20μg ethinylestradiol:

- Take most recent missed pill as soon as it is remembered.

- Discard any earlier missed pills.
- Take the remaining pills in the pack daily at the usual time (may mean taking two pills on the same day – one on remembering and one at the usual time; sometimes this may be the same time).
- Use condoms or abstain from sex until seven pills have been taken in a row. And:
  - If pills missed in first week of cycle (effectively extending the pill-free interval) and had unprotected sex in pill-free interval or in first week, consider emergency contraception.
  - If pills missed in third week of cycle, finish the current pack and start a new pack on the next day, thereby omitting the pill-free interval (avoids the need for emergency contraception).

If using everyday regimens and any inactive pills are missed, discard the missed inactive pills and then continue taking one pill per day.

Diarrhoea and vomiting

Vomiting up to two hours after taking an oral contraceptive can interfere with absorption, as can very severe diarrhoea. If vomiting occurs within two hours, take another active pill. Pill taking should be maintained during the illness, if possible. If severe vomiting or diarrhoea continues for two days or more, follow procedures for missed pills.

Travel

The risk of DVT may be increased among COC users during travel that involves prolonged immobility (perhaps five hours or more). The risk may be reduced by exercising during the journey, maintaining good hydration and, possibly, by the use of graduated compression stockings.

Surgery

COCs should be stopped (and adequate alternative contraception provided) four weeks before:

- Major elective surgery.
- Any surgery to the legs.
- Surgery that involves prolonged immobilisation of the lower limb.

Restart on the first day of the next period occurring at least two weeks after full mobilisation. If discontinuation is not possible (for example, emergency surgery), use thromboprophylaxis (heparin and graduated compression stockings). Minor surgery of short duration (for example, laparoscopic sterilisation or tooth extraction) does not need these procedures. These precautions are not necessary for users of progestogen-only contraceptives.

Concomitant use of other drugs

Short-term use of a liver enzyme-inducing drug (for example, barbiturates, carbamazepine, griseofulvin, modafinil, nelfinavir, nevirapine, oxcarbazepine, phenytoin, primidone, rifabutin, rifampicin, ritonavir, topiramate): needs use of a COC containing at least 50 micrograms of ethinylestradiol. Additional contraceptive protection should be used until four weeks after the liver-inducing enzyme is stopped. Short-term use of a broad-spectrum *antibiotic* (amoxycillin, ampicillin, augmentin, tetracycline and broad spectrum cephalosporin) needs extra contraception while taking the drug and for at least seven days after stopping. If these seven days run beyond the end of the packet, the next packet should be started immediately without a break (in the case of ED brands, omit the inactive pills). Rifampicin and rifabutin are such powerful liver enzyme-inducing drugs that even if the course lasts for less than seven days (for example, two days to eliminate carriage of meningococcus), extra contraception is needed until four weeks after stopping.

NB. Co-trimoxazole and erythromycin do not affect contraceptive cover – if anything they increase the blood levels of ethinylestradiol, although not dangerously so.

Long-term use of a liver enzyme-inducing drug: consider use of another contraceptive, such as an IUD, *especially if taking rifampicin or rifabutin*.

Long-term use of broad-spectrum antibiotics: the large bowel flora responsible for recycling estrogen develop antibiotic resistance after about three weeks, making extra contraception no longer necessary unless there is a change to a different antibiotic. Additional precautions are also not needed if a woman has been using broad-spectrum antibiotics for more than three weeks and starts using a COC.

Other drugs: occasional reports have appeared suggesting that COCs influence the pharmacotherapeutic effect of other drugs (for example, analgesics, antidepressants, benzodiazepines, B-blockers, corticosteroids, hypoglycaemic drugs, oral anticoagulants and theophylline). The documentation level regarding these interactions varies from 'possible' to 'probable'. So far, however, there is no evidence to suggest clinically significant effects which require the adjustment of the dose or prescription of an alternative medication[24,25].

Combined contraceptive patch

Description

A weekly contraceptive patch, usually worn on the buttock, lower abdomen or upper outer arm, delivering 20μg ethinylestradiol and 150μg norelgestromin per 24 hours. Main effects: prevention of ovulation; changes to cervical mucus making it hostile to sperm penetration; thinning of endometrium to prevent implantation.

Advantages

- Highly effective, non-intercourse related reversible contraceptive.
- Comparable safety and efficacy as COCs.
- May be useful for women who have difficulty remembering to take a daily COC.
- Not affected by diarrhoea or vomiting.

Disadvantages

- Similar adverse effect profile as COCs, with effects frequently decreasing with longer durations of use.
- Sometimes causes skin reactions to patch.
- May be visible.
- May be less effective in women heavier than 90kg.
- Relatively expensive; some authorities advise restricting use to women who are likely to comply poorly with COCs.
- Does not protect against STIs.

Do not use with these conditions (◉)
As for COCs (page 78).

Use cautiously with these conditions (▽)
As for COCs (page 79).

Broadly usable with these conditions (☼)
As for COCs (page 80)

Initial assessment before patch use

A careful personal and family medical history with particular attention to cardiovascular risk factors, and an accurate blood pressure measurement is sufficient for most women[26]. Further assessment is needed only if a relevant personal or family history is disclosed, or the blood pressure is elevated. In general, patches are broadly usable when there is one risk factor for venous thrombosis (for example, family history, obesity, long-term immobilisation, varicose veins) or arterial disease (for example, family history, diabetes, hypertension, smoking, age over 35, obesity, migraine). If there are two or more risk factors, use more cautiously or avoid use (depending on severity of the combining factors). Routine screening by means of physical examination (including breast and bimanual pelvic examination), urine or blood tests should not be a prerequisite for obtaining patches. Indeed, the routine use of such procedures can restrict accessibility to use of patches, as well as other methods of contraception.

Monitoring during usage

There is no consensus about how frequently follow-up visits should be. Many practitioners are likely to use the same practice as for COCs (see page 83). If a patch falls off, or starts to lose its adherence: reapply if still sticky, otherwise use a new patch. Adhesives or bandages should not be used to keep patches in place. If a patch has been off for less than 48 hours no additional contraception is needed; for longer periods (or where the user is uncertain) stop the current cycle, apply the first patch from a new cycle (making this 'change day' one of the new cycle) and use additional contraception for the next seven days.

If the last patch is left on beyond day 22 of the cycle, remove it when remembered and start the new cycle as usual on day one of the next cycle (that is, shorten the patch-free interval). No additional contraception is needed in these circumstances.

Delayed application of patch

If the first day of the next cycle is missed (that is, application of first patch in the next cycle delayed), contraception is lost. Apply the first patch of the new cycle when remembered, make this 'change day' one of the new cycle, and use additional contraception for the first seven days of the new cycle. If intercourse occurred during the extended patch-free period, consider the need for emergency contraception.

If the application of the second or third patch in a cycle is delayed beyond 'change day' eight or 15 respectively, and the delay is less than 48 hours, apply a new patch immediately and change the next patch on the normal change day; extra contraception is not needed. If the delay is more than 48 hours, stop the current cycle, apply the first patch from a new cycle (making this 'change day' one of the new cycle) and use additional contraception for the next seven days.

Concomitant use of other drugs

Liver enzyme-inducing drugs (see COC section, page 85 for details) may reduce the effectiveness of contraceptive patches. Use additional contraception while taking liver enzyme-inducing drugs and for four weeks afterwards. Women using liver enzyme-inducing drugs (including St John's wort) long-term, should consider changing to another method of contraception. Some antibacterials may affect the effectiveness of patches (see COC section on page 85, for details). Use additional contraception while taking the antibacterial and for seven days afterwards; if this period extends beyond the first three (active treatment) weeks of a contraceptive cycle, eliminate the patch-free week by starting a new cycle immediately.

Progestogen-only pills (POPs)

Description

Daily dose of oral progestogen which works, for most products, by making the cervical mucus hostile to sperm penetration, as well as prevention of ovulation in some cycles and endometrial effects. Contraceptive effects on cervical mucus thought to occur by 48 hours of POP use. The POP containing 75μg desogestrel inhibits ovulation in 97 per cent of cycles.

Advantages

- Effective, non-intercourse related, reversible.
- Can often be used by women with conditions which preclude the use of COCs.
- Can be used as an alternative to COCs before major surgery, before all surgery to the legs, or before surgery that involves prolonged immobilisation of a lower limb.
- Does not interfere with breastfeeding.

Disadvantages

- Requires consistent use every day, therefore not useful for forgetful users.
- Menstrual irregularity, from amenorrhoea to heavier more frequent periods; unpredictable and variable even in long-term users.
- Breast tenderness, often transient.
- Effect may be diminished in heavy women (arbitrarily defined as over 70kg) using levonorgestrel or norethisterone POPs (the evidence is uncertain, and does not relate to the desogestrel POP, but this should be discussed with the

woman. If risk of pregnancy unacceptable double the dose of POP or use the desogestrel POP).

- Hormonal contraceptives containing progestogen only have not been widely used, but the pattern of risk of breast cancer with time since last use appears to be similar to that found for COCs[27].

- Does not protect against STIs.

Do not use with these conditions (◉)

- Pregnancy.

- Current breast cancer.

Use cautiously with these conditions (▽)

- Gestational trophoblastic neoplasia, while hCG levels are abnormal (no restriction once levels become normal).

- Ischaemic heart disease, *if diagnosis occurs during use*.

- Stroke, *if occurs during use*.

- Migraine with aura, *if onset occurs during use*.

- Breast cancer: past history with no evidence of current disease for at least five years.

- Active viral hepatitis.

- Severe (decompensated) liver cirrhosis.

- Liver tumours: benign or malignant.

- Use of drugs which induce liver enzymes (for example, barbiturates, carbamazepine, modafinil, oxcarbazepine, phenytoin, primidone, rifabutin, rifampicin, topiramate and use of complementary medicines such as St John's wort).

Broadly usable with these conditions (☼)

- Past ectopic pregnancy (POP use actually reduces the risk of ectopic pregnancy, because ovulation is supressed in many POP users (especially those using desogestrel POPs), but other methods with more consistent suppression of ovulation (for example, COC, DMPA) may be preferable).

- Multiple risk factors for arterial disease (such as older age, smoking, diabetes and hypertension).

- Hypertension: controlled with vascular disease.

- Current or past history of DVT/PE.
- Known thrombogenic mutations (for example, Factor V Leiden, Prothrombin mutation, Protein S, Protein C and Antithrombin deficiencies).
- Major surgery with prolonged immobilisation.
- Ischaemic heart disease, *if diagnosis occurred before use*.
- Stroke, *if occurred before use*.
- Known hyperlipidaemia.
- Migraine: current problem without aura, *if onset occurs during use*; current problem with aura, *if onset occurred before use*; or past problem with aura.
- Diabetes with or without vascular disease.
- Breast disease: undiagnosed mass.
- Breast cancer: carrier of gene mutations known to be associated with elevated risk (for example, BRCA 1).
- Unexplained vaginal bleeding (important to exclude serious underlying illness, especially before starting POP).
- Abnormal vaginal bleeding patterns: irregular without heavy bleeding, or with heavy or prolonged bleeding (including regular patterns).
- Functional ovarian cysts causing pain.
- HIV positive, *if receiving anti-retroviral therapy*.
- AIDS and using HAART.
- Gallbladder/biliary tract disease, including asymptomatic disease.
- History of COC-related cholestasis.
- Mild (compensated) liver cirrhosis.
- Inflammatory bowel disease (includes ulcerative colitis and Crohn's disease).
- Raynaud's disease: secondary with lupus anticoagulant.
- Antiretroviral therapy (consult local HIV specialist or refer to www.hiv-druginteractions.org).

Initial assessment before POP use

A careful personal and family medical history with particular attention to cardiovascular risk factors, and an accurate blood pressure measurement is sufficient for most women. Further assessment is needed only if a relevant personal or family history is disclosed, or the blood pressure is elevated. Routine screening by means of physical examination (including breast and bimanual pelvic examination), urine or blood tests should not be a prerequisite for obtaining POPs. Indeed, the routine use of such procedures can restrict accessibility to use of POPs, as well as other methods of contraception.

POPs can be started up to and including day five without the need for additional contraception (otherwise use extra contraception for two days). Most POPs need to be taken within three hours of the same time each day; those with desogestrel within 12 hours. If changing from another hormonal method: can start POP immediately without the need for additional contraception, *provided that* the user has been using previous method consistently and correctly, and it is reasonably certain that the woman is not pregnant.

After childbirth and not breastfeeding: from day 21 after delivery; after three weeks and menstrual cycles *not* returned – start at any time if reasonably certain not pregnant (with additional contraceptive protection or abstinence from sex for two days); after three weeks and menstrual cycle returned – start as per any other woman with a menstrual cycle.

After childbirth and breastfeeding: if between six weeks and six months post-partum and menstrual cycle not returned – start at any time (with no additional contraception needed if fully or near fully breastfeeding); if more than six weeks post-partum and menstrual cycle returned – start as per any other woman with a menstrual cycle.

Monitoring during usage

There is no consensus about how frequently the follow-up visits need to be. The Faculty of Family Planning and Reproductive Health Care has stated that up to 12 months' supply of POP can be given at first and subsequent visits[28]. Many practitioners, however, would arrange an initial follow-up visit after one to three months of use to enquire about side effect or discuss problems. POPs do not appear to affect blood pressure in previously normotensive women, but may cause a small rise in women who have previously experienced blood pressure increases while using COCs. Given the simplicity and cheapness of the procedure, we recommend the monitoring of the blood pressure at the initial follow-up visit and annually thereafter. There is no need for other screening procedures simply because a woman is using POPs.

Broad-spectrum antibiotics do not affect POPs.

Missed POPs

A POP is regarded as 'missed' if taken more than three hours late, apart from the desogestrel-containing POP, Cerazette, which is regarded as 'missed' if taken more than 12 hours late. If a POP is missed, women should be told to take it as soon as they remember and to take their next pill at the usual time. This may mean that two pills are taken in one day. This is not harmful. If the pill was more than three hours overdue (or 12 hours for Cerazette) women are not protected. Continue normal pill taking but women must also use another method, such as the condom, for the next two days.

Emergency contraception should be considered if unprotected intercourse occurs when one or more POP has been missed or was taken more than three hours late.

Diarrhoea and vomiting

Vomiting up to two hours after taking a POP, or cases of very severe diarrhoea, may affect its absorption. If vomiting within two hours occurs, take another active pill. Continue taking pills at usual time if possible, despite discomfort. If severe vomiting or diarrhoea continues for two or more days, follow procedures for missed pills.

Barrier methods

Description

Various devices of different materials used by women and men to provide a physical barrier between the ejaculate and the female genital tract. Efficiency can be increased by the simultaneous use of spermicides for diaphragms and caps. Additional spermicide is not recommended with condoms. Spermicides used alone are not usually recommended, although they may be sufficiently effective in women when fertility is decreased, for example, during the climacteric.

Advantages

Contraceptive
- Readily available.
- Reasonable efficiency if used properly.
- May be preferred by couples who have infrequent intercourse, especially those wishing to have a 'more natural' form of birth control.
- Important adjunct when oral contraceptives are forgotten or of reduced efficacy (for example, during use of some antibiotics).

Non-contraceptive
- Useful protection against STIs (especially condoms, but not spermicides).
- Does not interfere with breastfeeding.

NB. Nonoxinol-9 has not been found to protect against STIs such as gonorrhoea or chlamydia, and it may increase the risk of HIV infection when used frequently by women at high risk of infection.

Disadvantages
- Reliant on user for effectiveness, intercourse-related.
- Often disliked because of aesthetics, reduced sensitivity during intercourse (with latex condoms).

Do not use with these conditions (◉)
- Any condition where pregnancy would be totally unacceptable to the user (use a more effective method).
- Spermicides should not be used if at high risk of getting an STI, including HIV (repeated and/or high doses of spermicide may cause vaginal wall abrasions, increasing the risk of transmission).

Use cautiously with these conditions (▽)
- HIV positive, irrespective of whether receiving anti-retroviral therapy (concern with use of spermicides associated with diaphragm use rather than the diaphragm itself).
- AIDS and using HAART (concern with use of spermicides associated with diaphragm use rather than the diaphragm itself).
- High risk of AIDS (concern with use of spermicides associated with diaphragm use rather than the diaphragm itself).
- History of toxic shock syndrome (diaphragm and contraceptive sponge).
- Irritation or sensitivity to latex condoms/diaphragms (silicone condoms and diaphragms exist).

Broadly usable with these conditions (☼)
- Parity (parous diaphragm users have a higher risk of failure than nulliparous users).

- Structural valvular or congenital heart disease, *if complicated* (diaphragm users: risk of urinary tract infection may increase risk of developing subacute bacterial endocarditis).
- CIN awaiting treatment (spermicide or cap not recommended).
- Cervical cancer awaiting treatment (spermicide or cap not recommended).
- Recurrent urinary tract infections in diaphragm users (use a smaller cervical cap instead).

Monitoring during usage
Diaphragm/cap users need to be checked for correct size every 12 months, if weight changes by more than 3kg or after delivery, abortion or miscarriage.

NB. Oil-based products, such as petroleum jelly (Vaseline), baby oil and oil-based vaginal and rectal preparations can damage latex (but not polyurethane) condoms and diaphragms, affecting both their contraceptive and STI-protective properties.

Natural family planning/fertility awareness

Description
Variety of methods to recognise or predict the timing of ovulation, in order to identify the fertile period:

- Calendar method.
- Temperature method.
- Cervical mucus method.
- Sympto-thermal/multiple index method.
- Fertility devices (for example, Persona)

The sympto-thermal method is the most effective (80 to 98 per cent effective) because it combines more than one indicator of fertility. With all fertility awareness methods, including Persona, careful adherence to the guidelines is important to ensure success.

Women should be advised that the first (pre-ovulatory) phase of reduced fertility is less 'safe', *however identified,* than the second (post-ovulatory) phase; greater efficacy can be achieved by restricting unprotected intercourse to the latter phase.

Advantages
- No known physical side effects.

- Non-intercourse related.

- May be only acceptable contraceptive for some with religious or personal beliefs which prevent using other methods of birth control.

- Once learnt does not need regular follow-up.

- Can be used to plan pregnancy as well as prevent conception.

Disadvantages
- Requires commitment from both partners.

- For most success, teaching requires specialist knowledge from natural family planning teachers.

- Requires careful observation and record keeping, with documentation of a number of cycles before ovulation can be reliably predicted.

- Fertility devices (Persona) are expensive to buy and use.

- Does not protect against STIs.

Breastfeeding (lactational amenorrhoea method – LAM)

Breastfeeding is a recognised effective contraceptive (98 per cent) provided that:

- the woman is fully or almost fully breast-feeding (that is, using no milk substitutes and feeding on demand day and night), *and*

- the baby is less than six months old, *and*

- menstruation has not returned.

As soon as any of these conditions change, alternative methods of contraception should be started.

Emergency contraception

Hormonal emergency contraception

Description

1.5 mg levonorgestrel taken as a single dose as soon as possible after first act of unprotected intercourse. Most effective when taken as soon as possible after unprotected intercourse; ideally within 12 hours and no later than 72 hours (licensed use) or 120 hours (unlicensed use).

Advantages

- Highly effective contraceptive (if taken within 24 hours of unprotected intercourse, prevents up to 95 per cent of pregnancies expected to occur if no emergency contraception had been used; if taken 72 hours afterwards prevents up to 58 per cent of expected pregnancies).
- Useful back-up for those who have had unprotected intercourse, including rape victims.
- Available free from a wide range of health service providers.
- Can be purchased without prescription from pharmacies and some privately run clinics such as bpas and Marie Stopes.

NB. Providing supplies in advance increases usage after unprotected intercourse without affecting use of routine contraception.

Disadvantages

- Some women experience nausea, headaches, dizziness, tiredness, breast tenderness and abdominal pain.

Do not use with these conditions (◉)

- Pregnancy.
- Current hepatocellular jaundice (consider IUD).
- Sickle cell crisis (consider IUD).

Use cautiously with these conditions (▽)

- Migraine with aura occurring at time of request for emergency contraception.

NB. Many authorities would place the above in the 'do not use' section.

Broadly usable with these conditions (☼)

- Using a liver enzyme-inducing drug (in which case increase the progestogen dose by 50 per cent or use IUD). No need to increase the dose for non-enzyme inducing antibiotics. Women who are offered an increased dose of levonorgestrel should be told that this use is outside the product licence.

Initial assessment before use

The history should include details of the last menstrual period, length of menstrual cycle, timing of all inadequately protected intercourse in this cycle (to ensure that the *first* episode of unprotected intercourse occurred less than 72 (120) hours previously), history of migraine with aura. The consultation is usually a useful opportunity to review continuing contraceptive needs and other aspects of sexual health.

Women should be advised that their next period may be earlier or later than usual, and that hormonal contraception can be continued or started immediately, otherwise they should use a barrier method of contraception (or abstain from intercourse) until the next period. If vomiting occurs within three hours of taking, give a replacement dose, possibly with an antiemetic such as domperidone (10mg).

Monitoring after usage
Many practitioners offer women a follow-up appointment at three to four weeks, as well as advising them to come sooner if they develop lower abdominal pain or heavy bleeding, or there are any other concerns such as ectopic pregnancy. If the next menstrual period is abnormally light, short or absent, pregnancy should be suspected. It should be managed as any other unintended pregnancy, since the pregnancy would not have been exposed to the emergency hormones which were given pre-implantation.

Copper IUD

Description
Insertion of copper IUD (that is, not hormone releasing) up to five days after earliest ovulation, calculated from woman's shortest likely cycle.

Advantages
- Most effective available method (two failures in 1300 insertions)[29].
- Offers continuing contraception, but if not appropriate can be removed at next menses.
- Useful when hormonal emergency contraception has induced vomiting, and replacement dose not sufficient to provide adequate cover.
- Useful if multiple exposure.
- Useful if migraine with aura, jaundice or sickle cell crisis.

Disadvantages
- Pain.
- Bleeding.
- Risk of infection.

Do not use with these conditions (◉)
- Pregnancy.
- As for IUDs generally (see page 73).

Use cautiously with these conditions (∇)
- As for IUDs generally (see page 74).

Broadly usable with these conditions (☼)
- As for IUDs generally (see page 74).

Initial assessment before insertion

The history should include details of the last menstrual period, length of menstrual cycle, timing of all inadequately protected intercourse in this cycle (to ensure that the insertion is within five days of ovulation) and aspects of history required to ensure the safe insertion of an IUD. The consultation is usually a useful opportunity to review continuing contraceptive needs and other aspects of sexual health. Ideally all women should be screened for STIs, and antibiotic cover considered (see page 75).

Monitoring during usage

Many practitioners offer women a follow-up appointment at three to four weeks, as well as advising them to come sooner if they develop lower abdominal pain or heavy bleeding, or there are any other concerns. If the next menstrual period is abnormally light, short or absent, pregnancy should be suspected. It should be managed as any other unintended pregnancy. If the woman wishes to continue with the pregnancy, the IUD should be removed to reduce the risk of miscarriage.

PERMANENT METHODS

Female sterilisation

Description

Occlusion of the fallopian tubes by a variety of surgical techniques (most commonly, mechanical means such as tubal clips or rings; also diathermy or partial salpingectomy) using a variety of surgical approaches (most frequently laparoscopy, but also laparotomy or mini-laparotomy)[30].

Advantages

- Highly effective.

- Immediacy of effect.

- Permanent.

- Not reliant on the user for effect.

- Can remove the fear of pregnancy.

Disadvantages

- Requires a surgical procedure (usually under light general anaesthetic but can be under local anaesthetic).

- Sometimes fails (failure rate 1 in 200 (1 in 333–500 for Filshie Clip) with some events occurring some years after the sterilization, emphasising the need to warn women to mention that they have been sterilised if they subsequently develop pelvic pain; failure is more common in younger women; perhaps a third of such pregnancies are ectopic).

- Not necessarily reversible (success of reversal more likely if clips rather than another method used, and if the woman is younger. Pregnancies after reversal are also more likely to be ectopic).

- Can cause regret (appears to be more common if done at young age (under 30 years), at time of relationship difficulties, if partnership is child-free, if performed just after childbirth, abortion or miscarriage, or when ambivalent about whether to have the operation).

- Has been said to cause menstrual upset afterwards although the evidence is inconsistent and may be due to other factors such as stopping COCs which were masking menstrual problems.

Special precautions

In general, the medical precautions are those which exist for any woman requiring a light general anaesthetic. The operation may be technically more difficult in obese women (laparoscopic sterilisation) or women with certain gynaecological problems.

Initial assessment before the operation

Ideally both partners should be involved in the decision. Careful counselling is required about the operation's permanence, risk of failure (including risk of ectopic pregnancy), and reassurance about no clear evidence of adverse effect on menstrual pattern. Information that vasectomy is equally as effective, but quicker, safer and cheaper than female sterilisation, should also be given. The greater tendency for childless women, and those aged less than 30 years, to regret their decision, means that such women and their partners need particularly careful counselling. Contraceptive measures should be used up to the first menstrual period after the sterilisation.

Monitoring after operation

Apart from the usual post-operative care, no other measures are required. Signs of ectopic pregnancy should be sought if any periods are missed, light or scanty especially if associated with lower abdominal pain.

Male sterilisation

Description

Excision of a segment, and occlusion by ligature, cautery or clip of remaining, vas deferentia by a small incision or puncture of the scrotal skin.

Advantages

- Highly effective.

- Permanent.

- Safe and easy, usually can be done under local anaesthesia.

- Not reliant on the user for effect.

- Can remove the fear of pregnancy.

Disadvantages

- Not effective immediately (may take three to four months; clinics vary when they start testing for effect).

- Requires a surgical procedure.

- Sometimes fails (failure rate about 1 per 2,000: can occur some years after operation even in men who have previously had negative sperm counts).

- Not necessarily reversible (success of reversal depends on: method used; age of man (better in younger men); interval between sterilisation and reversal attempt (poor if more than ten years)).

- Can cause regret (appears to be more common if done at young age (under 30 years), if the partnership is child-free, if done at time of relationship difficulties, or when ambivalent about whether to have the operation).

- Short-term side effects of scrotal bruising and swelling (less with the 'no scalpel' technique).

- Sperm granuloma causing the formation of nodules can occur in up to 30 per cent of men after vasectomy; tenderness is rare and lesion rarely needs excision.

Anti-sperm antibodies have been reported in a large proportion of men after vasectomy, but these do not appear to be associated with increased auto-immune disease. Previous concerns that vasectomy increases the risk of cardiovascular disease have not been substantiated. Some studies have indicated that vasectomy increases the risk of prostatic and testicular cancer; findings which have been contradicted by other research. On the basis of existing biological and epidemiological evidence, any causal relationship between vasectomy and risk of prostate and testicular cancer is unproven and no changes in family planning policies concerning vasectomy are justified. It is important, however, to include discussion of the subject as part of the counselling, if only because future research is likely to attract media attention.

Special precautions
In general, there are few medical precautions for the operation. The operation may be technically more difficult in men with certain urological problems.

Initial assessment before the operation
Ideally both partners should be involved in the decision. Careful counselling about the operation's permanence and risk of failure is required. The greater tendency for men who are childless, or aged less than 30 years, to regret their decision, means that such men and their partners need particularly careful counselling.

Monitoring after operation
Other contraceptive methods should be used until a negative semen sample has been obtained[31].

Key messages

- The primary care team has the opportunity to deliver high quality contraceptive services.

- Decisions about the choice of contraceptive involve a number of issues including method effectiveness, perceived safety, recognised contraindications, acceptability, ease of use, and availability.

- Users of contraceptive services need up-to-date, comprehensive information about each method of contraception.

- In delivering a high quality service, the primary care team needs to ensure that the full range of contraceptive methods is available, even if this requires referral to another agency.

- In the end, confidence in the services provided depends on the provision and standard of care. If users feel confident and supported, they are more likely to use their chosen method of contraception successfully.

Table 3.1:

Conditions requiring particular consideration when choosing a reversible method of contraception

Condition	Inj	Imp	IUS	IUD	COC/patch	POP	Bar
Age <18	☆						
<20							
≥35			☆	☆	◉a		
>45	☆						
Non smoker >35					☆ ▽a /☆		
Smoker <35							
≥35 and:							
i) < 15 cigarettes a day					◉a ▽		
ii) ≥ 15 cigarettes a day					◉		
iii) stopped smoking < 1 year ago					▷		
iv) stopped smoking ≥1 year ago					☆		
Obesity:							
i) body mass index (BMI) 30 to 34 kg/m²					☆		
ii) body mass index (BMI) 35 to 39 kg/m²					▷		
iii) body mass index (BMI) ≥40 kg/m²					◉		
Parous							☆b
Pregnancy	◉	◉	◉	◉	◉	◉	
Puerperal sepsis			◉	◉			
Questionable fertility for whatever reason	☆	☆	☆	☆			

THE HANDBOOK OF SEXUAL HEALTH IN PRIMARY CARE

Condition	Inj	Imp	IUS	IUD	COC/patch	POP	Bar
Post-partum: < 6 weeks (fully or almost fully breastfeeding)	☼				◉		
6 weeks to < 6months (fully or almost fully breastfeeding)					▷		
6 weeks to < 6 months (medium to low partial breastfeeding)					☼		
Post-partum (including post-caesarian section), irrespective of breastfeeding practices: <4 weeks			▷	▷			
≥4 weeks							
Post-abortion: Immediate post-septic abortion			◉	◉			
Up to 24 weeks pregnancy			☼	☼			
Gestational trophoblastic neoplasia: hCG normal	▷	▷					
hCG abnormal			◉	◉	◉	▷	
Multiple risk factors for arterial cardiovascular disease	▷	☼	☼		◉a / ▷c	☼	
Hypertension: controlled without vascular problems	☼	☼			▷		
controlled with vascular problems	▷		☼		◉	☼	
Consistently elevated blood pressure levels: systolic 140–159 or diastolic 90–94 mm Hg					▷		
systolic ≥160 or diastolic ≥95 mm Hg	☼				◉		
History of high blood pressure during pregnancy					☼		

Condition	Inj	Imp	IUS	IUD	COC/patch	POP	Bar
Deep vein thrombosis/pulmonary thrombosis:							
personal history	☆	☆	☆		◉	☆	
current disease	▷	▷	▷	▷	◉	☆	
known thrombogenic mutations	☆	☆	☆		◉	☆	
major surgery: with prolonged immobilisation	☆	☆	☆		◉	☆	
without prolonged immobilisation					☆		
long-term immobilisation					▷		
family history: first degree relative aged <45 years					▷		
first degree relative ≥ 45 years					☆		
Varicose veins (with no definite history of DVT)							
Superficial venous thrombosis:							
superficial thrombophlebitis					☆		
varicose veins					☆		
Ischaemic heart disease: current/personal history	▷	▽d/☆e	▽d/☆e		◉	▽d/☆e	
Structural heart disease (valvular and congenital)							
uncomplicated			☆	☆	☆		
complicated			☆		◉		☆b
Stroke: current/personal history	▷	▽d/☆e	☆		◉	▽d/☆e	
Known hyperlipidaemia	☆	☆	☆		▽a/☆	☆	

Condition	Inj	Imp	IUS	IUD	COC/patch	POP	Bar
Headaches:							
non-migrainous (mild or severe)	☆ed	☆ed	☆ed		☆d	☆d	
migraine without aura, age < 35 years	☆ed	☆ed	☆ed		☆e/▽d	☆d	
migraine without aura, age ≥35 years	▽d/☆e	▽d/☆e	▽d/☆e		◙d/▽e	▽d/☆e	
migraine with aura, any age	☆	☆	☆		▽	☆	
past history of migraine with aura at any age							
Diabetes (insulin and non-insulin dependent):							
without vascular problems	☆	☆	☆		☆	☆	
with vascular problems or > 20 yrs duration	▽	☆	☆		◙a/▽	☆	
Breast disease: undiagnosed mass	☆	☆	☆		▽e/☆d	☆	
Breast cancer:							
current	◙	◙	◙		◙	◙	
past and no evidence of disease for 5 years	▽	▽	▽		▽	▽	
carriers of known associated gene mutations (eg BRCA 1)	☆	☆	☆		▽	☆	
Vaginal bleeding:							
unexplained (before evaluation)	▽	▽	◙e/☆d	◙e/☆d	☆	☆	
irregular *without* heavy loss	☆	☆	◙e/☆d	◙e/☆d	☆	☆	
heavy/prolonged loss (+/- irregular)	☆	☆	☆d	☆		☆	
with severe dysmenorrhoea	☆	☆		☆			
Cervix: carcinoma-in-situ (awaiting treatment)	☆	☆	☆	◙e/☆d	☆	☆	☆fg
cancer (awaiting treatment)	☆	☆	◙e/☆d	◙e/☆d	☆	☆	☆fg
Ovarian: cancer			▽e/☆d	▽e/☆d			
functional cysts causing pain						☆	
Endometrial cancer			◙e/☆d	◙e/☆d			

Condition	Inj	Imp	IUS	IUD	COC/patch	POP	Bar
Uterine fibroids: distorting uterine cavity			◉	◉			
Anatomic abnormalities :							
severely distorting uterine cavity, < 5.5mm size			◉	◉			
interfering with insertion, eg cervical stenosis			☼	☼			
Endometriosis				☼			
Pelvic inflammatory disease:							
past without subsequent pregnancy			☼ / ◉e/☼d	☼ / ◉e/☼d			
current or within 3 months			◉e/☼d				
Sexually transmissible infection:							
current or within 3 months			◉e/☼d	◉e/☼d			◉g
vaginitis without purulent cervicitis			☼	☼			
increased risk			▽e/☼d	▽e/☼d			◉g
HIV/AIDS:							
HIV +ve not using anti-retroviral therapy		☼	☼	☼			▽b
HIV +ve and using anti-retroviral therapy		☼	☼	☼			▽b
AIDS and using HAART	☼		☼	☼	☼	☼	▽b
increased risk HIV/AIDS			☼	☼	☼	☼	◉g / ▽b
Pelvic tuberculosis			◉e / ▽d	◉e / ▽d			
Toxic shock syndrome: past history							▽b
Urinary tract infection: recurrent							☼b
Gallbladder/biliary tract disease: symptomatic	☼	☼	☼		▽	☼	
asymptomatic	☼	☼	☼		☼	☼	

Condition	Inj	Imp	IUS	IUD	COC/patch	POP	Bar
Cholestasis: pregnancy-related	☼	☼	☼		☼	☼	
past COC-related					▷		
Viral hepatitis: active	▷	▷	▷		◉	▷	
Liver cirrhosis: mild (compensated)	☼	☼	☼		▷	☼	
severe (decompensated)	▷	▷	▷		◉	▷	
Wilson's disease				◉			
Liver tumours: benign or malignant	▷	▷	▷		◉	▷	
Inflammatory bowel disease					☼	☼	
Thalassaemia				☼			
Sickle cell *disease* (not trait – which is not affected by choice)				☼	☼		
Iron deficiency anaemia				☼			
Raynaud's disease: primary	☼	☼	☼		☼		
secondary without lupus anticoagulant							
secondary with lupus anticoagulant					◉	☼	
Allergy to: copper				◉			
latex							▷

Condition	Inj	Imp	IUS	IUD	COC/patch	POP	Bar
Drug interactions :							
Drugs which affect liver enzymes:							
anti-infectives (griseofulvin, rifampicin, rifabutin)		▷			▷	▷	
anti-convulsants (barbituates, carbamazepine, oxcarbazepine, phenytoin, primidone, topiramate)		▷			▷	▷	
complementary medicines such as St John's wort		▷			▷	▷	
Others (modafinil)		▷			☼	▷	
Non-liver enzyme inducing antibiotics		☼			☼	☼	
Highly active antiretroviral therapy (HAART)	☼		▽e / ☼d	▽e / ☼d	☼	☼	
Strong immunosuppressives (but corticosteroids alright)			◎	◎			

◎ Do not use with these conditions.

▽ Use cautiously with these conditions.

☼ Broadly usable with these conditions.

a. If other arterial risk factors present, especially if severe.

b. Diaphragm users.

c. User <35 years.

d. If occurs during use.

e. If known about before use.

f. Cap should not be used, no restriction for diaphragm use.

g. Spermicides only.

Table 3.2:

Efficacy of contraceptive methods

Methods that have no 'user' failure	Percentage per 100 women per year
Contraceptive injection	Over 99% effective
Implant	Over 99% effective
Intrauterine system (IUS)	Over 99% effective in first year (over 98% over 5 years)
Intrauterine device (IUD)	Around 99% effective (depending in IUD type)
Female sterilisation	Over 99% effective, lifetime failure rate 1 in 200 (depending on method used)
Male sterilisation (vasectomy)	Over 99% effective, lifetime failure rate of about 1 in 2,000
Methods that have 'user' failure *	
Combined oral contraceptive	Up to 99+% effective
Combined contraceptive patch	Up to 99+% effective
Progestogen-only oral contraceptive	Up to 99% effective
Male condom	Up to 98% effective
Female condom	Up to 95% effective
Diaphragm or cap + spermicide	Latex types: up to 92% to 96% effective Silicone caps less effective

Natural family planning:
    Sympto-thermal method
    New technologies (Persona)
	
	Up to 98% effective (if several fertility indictors used)
	Up to 94% effective

* *NB.* efficacy rates reflect the method when used absolutely correctly and consistently. Where methods are used less well, lower efficacy rates will occur.

Reproduced from the *Contraceptive Handbook*[32].

Table 3.3:

Risks of pregnancy with no contraception

Age of woman (years)	% per 100 women per year
< 40	80–90%
40	40–50%
45	10–20%
50+	0–5%

Figures from *Contraception Today*[33].

References

1. World Health Organisation. *Medical Eligibility Criteria for Contraceptive Use*, 3rd edition, Geneva: World Health Organization 2004.

2. *UK Medical Eligibility Criteria for Contraceptive Use*. To be published See http://www.ffprhc.org.uk

3. Hannaford P and Webb A. *Evidence-guided Prescribing of Combined Oral Contraceptives*: *Consensus Statement*, on behalf of participants at an international workshop, *Contraception*, vol 54, no 3, 1996, pp125–29.

4. Faculty of Family Planning and Reproductive Health Care (FFPRHC), *UK Selected Practice Recommendations for Contraceptive Use*. London: FFPRHC 2002.

5. Joint Formulary Committee. *British National Formulary 47*. British Medical Association and Royal Pharmaceutical Society of Great Britain 2004.

6. See note 1 above.

7. See note 2 above.

8. See note 4 above.

9. See note 5 above.

10. See note 4 above.

11. See note 5 above.

12. Guillebaud J. *Contraception Today*. London: Taylor and Francis 2003.

13. **fpa**. Contraceptive leaflets, updated regularly. **fpa**.

14. Guillebaud J. *Contraception – Your Questions Answered*. London: Churchill Livingstone 2004.

15. Glaiser A and Gebbie A (eds). *Handbook of Family Planning and Reproductive Health Care*. London: Churchill Livingstone 2000.

16. See note 13 above.

17. See note 4 above.

18. Collaborative Group on Hormonal Factors in Breast Cancer. Breast cancer and hormonal contraceptives: further results. *Contraception,* vol 54, no 3 (suppl), 1996, pp1–106S.

19. Medicines and Healthcare Products Regulatory Agency. *Updated Prescribing Advice on the Effect of Depo-provera Contraception on Bones*. London: MHRA 2004.

20. See note 18 above.

21. See note 3 above.

22. See note 4 above.

23. Faculty statement from the Clinical Effectiveness Unit on a new publication: *WHO Selected Practice Recommendations from Contraceptive Use* update. Missed pills: new recommendations. *Journal of Family Planning and Reproductive Health Care*, vol 31, no 2, 2005, pp153–55.

24. Geurts T, Goorissen E and Sitsen J (eds). *Summary of Drug Interactions with Oral Contraceptives*. Parthenon 1993; and refer to http://www.hiv-druginteractions.org

25. Faculty of Family Planning and Reproductive Health Care Guidance (April 2005) Drug interactions with hormonal contraception. *Journal of Family Planning and Reproductive Health Care*, vol 31, no 2, 2005, pp139–51.

26. See note 3 above.

27. See note 18 above.

28. See note 4 above.

29. See note 14 above.

30. Royal College of Obstetricians and Gynaecologists (RCOG). *Male and Female Sterilisation: Evidence-based Clinical Guideline* No 4, London: RCOG, 2004.

31. See note 30 above.

32. Belfield T. *Contraceptive Handbook.* **fpa** 1999.

33. See note 12.

Annex 1

EMERGENCY CONTRACEPTION GUIDANCE

Concrete Towers Practice

Leads[1]
- Dr Rose Green
- Ms Violet Brown

External reviewer[2]
- Dr X Pert

Aims
- to prevent unwanted pregnancy this cycle
- to prevent unwanted pregnancy in the future
- to increase awareness of STIs and how to avoid them in those at risk
- to increase detection of STIs in those at risk
- to provide a non-judgemental service.

Access and signposting[3]
Women can access emergency contraception (EC) by:
- seeing the GP in morning or evening surgery in the usual way
- asking for 'an emergency appointment with the nurse'
- accessing a primary care based sexual health outreach worker (SHOW)[4] directly
- NHS Walk-in centres (open every day of the year)
- Brook – for those age under 25 (every day except Sunday)
- sold in pharmacies for £25 if aged 16 or over (free to under 21's from participating pharmacies in scheme operated by some PCTs).

---

1. Appropriate clinical members of the team.
2. Usually a local specialist.
3. These options will differ considerably for different areas.
4. See Chapter 1 for an account of SHOW.

This service should be clearly promoted in ways which signal to patients that it is available, and how it can be accessed: moving message, practice leaflet, other posters and leaflets.

Promotion of emergency contraception (EC) can usefully occur at new registration, abortion referral consultations, condom provision and during many other consultations.

Emergency hormonal contraception (EHC)

Preparation
Levonorgestrel 1.5 mg tab

*Altered dose if patient taking **enzyme inducing medication** – increase by 50 per cent, that is, add a half tab or 0.75 mg tab.*

Timing
Can be given up to 120 hours (five days) after unprotected sexual intercourse (UPSI), the first 72 of which are within licence (see *IUCD for emergency contraception,* in this guidance, page 115). EHC can be used more than once in a cycle.

Effectiveness
Is not as effective at any stage as an intrauterine contraceptive device (IUCD)[5].

Prevents approximately:

- 95 per cent of pregnancies if given 0–24 hours after UPSI
- 85 per cent at 24–48 hours
- 58 per cent at 48–72 hours
- See *Unlicenced use of oral EC,* page 118, in this guidance, for 72–120 hours.

Should be given as a **single dose** (one 1.5mg tab).

The majority of women have their period within three days of the expected date.

Future contraceptive cover
The chosen contraceptive method **should be started at the time that emergency contraception is given** (and no more than 12 hours later if, for example, COC is to be resumed). This reduces the number of pregnancies that occur while awaiting

---

5.   This practice has chosen to use the abbreviation IUCD as opposed to IUD.

the next period. Longer acting contraceptives are most efficacious, for example implants. There is no evidence that hormonal contraceptive methods harm early pregnancies. An IUCD will act as emergency contraceptive *and* give long acting cover.

A pregnancy test should be arranged if the period does not occur by one week after it was expected. Women starting hormonal contraception at the time of EC should return for a pregnancy test if their period is absent, or shorter than normal.

Consider active follow-up **or** *SHOW referral for those at high risk.*
Record phone or other contact details.

STI risk

Risk of STI is in general higher in this group, although may be non-existent for some women: do a risk assessment. A chlamydia test should be offered then or in the near future, or in some cases, a full STI screen. Give advice on prevention of STIs, give condoms.

Consider active follow up **or** *SHOW referral for those at high risk.*
Record phone or other contact details.

Consider referring the following people for follow-up by SHOW:

- women under 18
- women of any age with a third request for EC in one year
- women who have chaotic use of contraception
- women who have had one or more abortions in the last three years.

IUCD for emergency contraception[6]

For those:

- who want most effective EC
- in whom oral EC is contraindicated
- who want it as ongoing contraception
- who have no contraindications to IUCD
- who choose IUCD EC
- with multiple exposure this cycle.

---

6. Please also refer to the practice IUCD clinical guidelines.

Device

Tsafe Cu380A

Nova T 380s for difficult fittings (slightly slimmer) and so consider for those who are absolutely sure they only want it for EC and not ongoing contraception (although if they then change their minds it can be left in situ).

Timing

Up to 120 hours after UPSI

Up to and within 5 days of *earliest* predicted ovulation (EPO is usually taken as 14 days before next period, *as long as LMP is known and cycle is regular*).

STI risk

Risk of STI is in general higher in this group, although may be non-existent for some women. In general prophylactic antibiotics *and* chlamydia testing should be provided in all but exceptional circumstances.

In some cases a full STI screen should be conducted or arranged.

Give advice on prevention of STIs, give condoms.

*Consider active follow-up **or** SHOW referral for those at high risk.
Record phone or other contact details.*

Follow-up

*Mark computer record for active follow up in two to three weeks.
Consider SHOW referral.
Record phone or other contact details.*

Requires follow up to:

- IUCD check if continuing, at six weeks
- remove with/after period if desired only for EC
- exclude pregnancy (including ectopic) if period does not occur.

Some women may wish to switch to another contraceptive method, which should be done seven days before removal of IUCD and after the first period with IUCD in situ has commenced.

*Consider active follow-up **or** SHOW referral for those at high risk.
Record phone or other contact details.*

Consider referring the following people for follow up by SHOW:

- women under 18
- women of any age with a third request for EC in one year
- women who have chaotic use of contraception
- women who have had one or more abortions in the last three years.

Missed or late contraception and EC

COC[7]

If missed pills (more than 24 hours late) during **week three** of packet:

- skip pill-free week (go straight on to next packet).

Also a back up method (for example, condoms), or abstinence, for seven days if the following number of pills are missed:

- 'two for 20' (that is, if two or more 20 mcg ethinylestradiol pills are missed)
- 'three for 30' (that is, if three or more 30–35 mcg ethinylestradiol pills are missed).

May need EC if fail to abstain/use condoms after missing pills.

POP

If one or more pills are missed *or* pill taken more than three hours late and extra precautions (for 48 hours) not taken, then EC indicated. For desogestrel POP (Cerazette) the interval for a late pill is longer – 12 hours – before EC is indicated (extra precautions again).

Contraceptive patch

If the patch *is not replaced*:

- up to day nine, replace patch (unless week three that is, patch-free interval)
- after day nine, use emergency contraception if UPSI has occurred, and additional contraception is needed for seven days.

If a patch *falls off*:

- up to 24 hours, replace patch
- after 24 hours (or if unsure) use emergency contraception if UPSI has occurred, and additional contraception is needed for seven days.

---

7. 'Faculty Statement from the CEU – Missed Pills: new recommendations'. April 2005.

If *new patch forgotten* after patch-free week:

- up to 48 hours delay, restart patch when remembered
- after 48 hours, use emergency contraception if UPSI has occurred and additional contraception is needed for seven days.

DMPA

Delayed DMPA:

- within 14 weeks of previous injection no extra precautions required, give next Depo if patient wants to continue
- consider EC if any sexual intercourse without barriers takes place after 14 weeks, care re: follow-up, risk of pregnancy and future contraceptive follow-up.

EC to cover IUCD removal

EC should be given if an IUCD or IUS has to be removed and patient has had sexual intercourse that is otherwise unprotected in the last seven days. Problems can be prevented if replacement contraception is started seven days before removal.

Unlicensed use of oral EC

Use of oral EC is currently unlicensed when used beyond 72 hours after UPSI. However its use in this way may be considered best practice under some circumstances. This unlicensed use of oral EC needs to be recorded (see checklist/ template). The 2002 WHO trial found effectiveness to be 50–60 per cent between 72 and 120 hours post UPSI *but* numbers were small.

Fraser Guidance	Not applicable	Criteria satisfied: Yes/No

LMP

UPSI/condom accident*	Date: _____	Time: __ Hours ago
Previous UPSI this cycle*	Yes/No	When
Liver disease	Yes/No	What
Recent medication	Yes/No	What
Recent GI Upset	Yes/No	When
Risk of STI	High/Moderate/None	

Contraception to date:

Contraceptive choice now:

No. times EC this year?	**No. abortions in last three years?**
IUCD discussed?	Yes/No
Condoms	Discussed Yes/No Given Yes/No

What might do if pregnant

Contact details/mobile

Explanation, management and follow-up: When/how to take

Action to take if vomiting occurs   Not teratogenic

What to expect re bleeding/plan for f/u for PT if period more than 7d late

Risk of pregnancy/symptoms of ectopic

F/U re STI?	**F/U re contraception?**
SHOW referral?	**Written info given:**

Give EHC stat in surgery*

Do script to replace stock and give to nurses

***Is use within licence?**	Yes/No If no, why:

---

8.   This section can form the basis of a computer template.

Chapter 4

PREGNANCY PLANNING

Tom Heyes

INTRODUCTION

This chapter aims to guide primary care practitioners who wish to work with patients before they become pregnant, in order to promote the best possible pregnancy outcomes. The developing field of preconception care has a limited amount of clinical evidence to support it. Many primary care teams do not devote much attention to the topic, believing that there is no great demand from patients, and that there is a lack of established practice[1]. However, sufficient evidence is available to indicate that significant health improvements could result from a programme of preconception care. It suggests that poor pregnancy outcomes, particularly low birth weight and prematurity, could be reduced and that there is a significant unmet demand for preconception care from those who are aware of its potential benefits.

OVERVIEW OF EVIDENCE

What determines pregnancy outcomes?

The main pregnancy outcomes of interest in the developed world are birthweight, pre-term birth, miscarriage, stillbirth and malformations. Also important are neurodevelopmental problems and allergies, and pregnancy complications such as pre-eclampsia and infections. In developing countries maternal mortality and morbidity have greater prominence.

Epidemiological research indicates a number of factors associated with a higher rate of adverse outcomes. They include low income and educational attainment, other indices of deprivation, smoking, the presence in the body of toxic substances including lead, cadmium, mercury and persistent organic poisons, use of drugs including alcohol and caffeine, and poor diet, particularly folate deficiency. Maternal health status indicated by measures such as height is an important determinant of birthweight, pointing to significant transgenerational effects on infant health[2].

Recent reviews of published work on nutritional and other interventions *during* pregnancy to prevent pre-term birth and low birthweight showed very little effectiveness[3,4,5].

A search of the published literature indicates that there has been little experimental research on preconception interventions. The use of folic acid as a supplement is supported by randomised controlled trial evidence[6] but the implementation even of this measure is incomplete[7,8]. The approach recommended here is therefore based mainly on epidemiological evidence and the opinion of practitioners.

The efforts of individual clinicians should be supplemented by other action, arguably more important and effective in the longer term, to reduce social inequalities and improve education generally[9]. Nutrition needs to be addressed by measures such as improving the availability of good quality food and the ability to purchase it, particularly in deprived areas. Some foods such as cereals are fortified with folic acid and this could be extended to include additional foods. More effective national action is needed to reduce smoking, particularly among young women.

THE CLINICAL APPROACH

Primary care practices will encounter both women and couples before a pregnancy in a number of different situations:

- those not considering or ambivalent about future pregnancy
- those contemplating their first pregnancy with no apparent risk factors
- those who have had good outcomes from previous pregnancies
- those who have had poor outcomes including infertility, miscarriages, pre-term births and low birthweight babies
- the presence of other known risk factors for problems in pregnancy such as greater maternal age, chronic diseases, specific genetic factors and exposure to hazards including smoking, drugs and occupational risks.

Each of these circumstances will require a modified approach to address the main perceived risks. Bear in mind that many pregnancies are 'unplanned', and that the planning process is complex and ambiguous. Advice can still be offered to people who are not currently planning a pregnancy. The outline given here can be adapted accordingly.

History-taking

- **Debriefing/narrative**. Ask about the woman's or couple's reproductive history. This is useful for indicating where future problems may occur. It will also help to establish a rapport and avoid insensitive questioning or advice. Some people have a traumatic story to relate – being listened to can have a therapeutic effect.

- **Obstetric history**. Losses, pre-term births, low birthweights and any other problems, including a history of haemolytic streptococcus Group B disease (see the RCOG guidance on www.rcog.org.uk). Infertility. Use of contraception. Frequency of intercourse. Menstrual pattern. Number of months of sexual activity without contraception when conception has not occurred. Any investigations carried out previously including tests for fertility, for urinary and genital infection and cervical cytology. Couples receiving assisted conception treatments may be particularly in need of preconception care. History of pelvic infections and surgery. Question sensitively about number of previous sexual partners as this has a bearing on the risk of infections being present and the need for infection screening (see Chapter 2).

- **Anxieties and strengths**. Attitude to pregnancy. There is often ambivalence about embarking on a pregnancy, and the couple may have different attitudes. There may be a desire for a baby but concerns over issues such as finances and careers can make this a difficult decision.

- **Relationships**. It may be appropriate to explore the couple's relationship in a non-judgemental manner. Women in many circumstances may wish to conceive, for instance those in a same-sex relationship or those who are post-menopausal. If there are difficulties within a couple's relationship, particularly if there is domestic violence, they are likely to be exacerbated by the stresses of pregnancy and childbirth. The team needs to decide how it will respond to all of these situations in the local context.

- **Smoking history**. If a smoker, assess readiness to quit.

- **Alcohol, drugs, prescribed, purchased and recreational**. Assess motivation to change. Obtain a detailed history of all medications used including those purchased over the counter. Recent evidence[10] implicates non-steroidal anti-inflammatory drugs as a cause of miscarriage.

- **Occupational and environmental hazards**. Ask about hobbies such as gardening and modelling as well as employment as these may include significant exposures to hazards such as pesticides and solvents without proper protection. Ask about exposure to lead, cadmium and mercury. Lead is the commonest hazard and now that it is not used in petrol the main domestic sources are old water piping and paint.

- **Genetics**. Availability of genetic information and testing is increasing. It may be necessary to obtain advice from a clinical geneticist for people with a family history of genetic disorders. Enquire whether the prospective parents belong to an ethnic group with a known genetic risk such as a haemoglobinopathy. In some communities it is appropriate to enquire about whether the couple have common ancestors or relatives.

- **Diet/exercise/relaxation/stress and hours of work**. Take a brief dietary history concentrating on the intake of the five major food groups – protein, complex carbohydrates, dairy products, fruit and vegetables, and sugars and fats. Essential fatty acids are also important and the consumption of fish has been shown to increase birthweight and possibly pregnancy duration[11]. A Body Mass Index (BMI) above or below the normal range increases the risk of a poor outcome. This enquiry may also detect people with eating disorders. Ask about the use of supplements, particularly folic acid. Find out if there are any other extreme features in the woman's lifestyle such as excessive exercise or very long hours of work.

- **Chronic diseases**. Ask about the presence of chronic diseases, particularly diabetes, epilepsy and thyroid disorders, allergies, and atopic status. The primary care practice is usually aware of these conditions.

- **Rubella and hepatitis**. Ask about immunisation status.

Examination and investigation

- Height, weight, BMI.

- If indicated, carry out a genital examination and take samples for infection screening (see Chapter 6).

- Test for Rubella immunity if status unknown. If risk factors exist or if local policy supports this, test also for hepatitis A, B and C, varicella and HIV.

Advice

Diet

Emphasise the value of five or more portions of fruit and vegetables a day for optimum intake of micronutrients. The nutrient content of fruit and vegetables is generally higher if they are fresh, raw or lightly cooked. Many women have a diet that is deficient in several nutrients[12] and this is not likely to be corrected by improving the diet for a few weeks or months prior to pregnancy. Hence, despite the lack of conclusive research-based evidence, a good quality multi-vitamin and mineral supplement can be advised. This should be suitable for use in pregnancy as standard supplements may contain too much Vitamin A which can be harmful. As a minimum, women should take a 400 microgram supplement of folic acid daily to reduce the risk of neural tube defects in the baby. This should be taken from the time they stop using contraception, until the twelfth week of pregnancy. For women who have previously had a baby with neural tube defects, or who are receiving anti-epileptic medication, a higher dose of 5 milligrams a day is recommended.

The intake of essential fatty acids by eating oily fish and seeds, or the oils extracted from them, should also be encouraged, though there are hazards from eating some fish because of the mercury content. Couples should avoid eating shark, swordfish and marlin and eat no more than one tuna steak a week (weighing about 140g cooked or 170g raw) or two medium-sized cans of tuna a week (with a drained weight of about 140g per can)[13].

Advise women about avoiding other hazards such as toxoplasma (contained in soiled cat litter and soil in the garden), listeria (in poorly cooked and stored food, soft cheeses and pâté) and salmonella (raw egg products). Consumption of liver products with their excessive vitamin A should also be limited[14]. If there appear to be problems, consider referral to a dietician for more detailed assessment and advice.

Social support
Consider interventions to develop the relationship, prepare for parenthood, and advise about benefits and employment rights.

Medical advice
Address identified risks including existing medical conditions and give appropriate advice about the risks to pregnancy. Diabetes and epilepsy pose particular problems and specialist advice should be taken before pregnancy, as excellent diabetic control improves the outcome greatly [15,16]. There are also hazards relating to anticonvulsant medications, which may need to be changed or stopped[17]. There is some evidence that allergies in infants can be prevented or reduced by measures taken during pregnancy, especially if there is a family history of atopy[18].

Any ongoing or intermittently used medication should be reviewed and the risks and benefits re-assessed in the light of the intended pregnancy. Some medications can be stopped or changed to safer ones. Refer to the British National Formulary (BNF) for advice about hazards of drugs in pregnancy. Most complementary therapies used can be considered safe, but couples should be advised to discuss the details with the therapist concerned. Women who may become pregnant should consult a qualified herbalist before taking any herbal medicines as some are contraindicated in pregnancy.

Live virus immunisations should be avoided in the month before conception for theoretical reasons, though in practice there is no evidence that this is harmful.

Environmental hazards

Prospective parents are often concerned about work stress and occupational hazards such as chemicals encountered in the workplace, or exposure to VDU screens. Suggest that they discuss with the responsible health and safety officer the fact that they are intending a pregnancy in order to ensure that all appropriate health and safety precautions are taken. Most working conditions do not appear to have major effects on pregnancy outcomes, but one study shows that the ability to control one's pace of work is correlated with better pregnancy health[19].

There is little hard evidence about adverse effects from VDU screens or other sources of electromagnetic radiation including mobile phones, microwave ovens and other domestic electrical devices such as electric blankets, vacuum cleaners and hairdryers[20], but there are theoretical grounds for considering them a hazard and so it may be prudent to minimise exposure.

Most X-ray examinations during pregnancy are considered low-risk but should only be carried out if there is clear benefit. Procedures that directly irradiate the fetus or that involve a higher dose of radiation, such as barium enemas, multiple-view lumbar spine examinations and CT scans have a higher risk, but may still be needed in certain circumstances[21].

Concerns have been raised about the use of mercury amalgam during dental treatment. While there is no clear evidence, UK advice currently is to avoid unnecessary placement or removal of mercury amalgam during pregnancy[22].

Sexual activity

Some couples may have false ideas about the frequency of intercourse required to conceive and can be reassured that most (84 per cent)[23] will do so within a year with unscheduled regular sex (two to three times a week) and that sex in early pregnancy is not harmful, unless it carries a risk of sexually transmissible infections (STIs). Education about fertility may be useful. If there are risk factors that can be improved such as smoking, obesity, or exposure to other significant hazards, it may be wise to use a readily reversible contraceptive method until this is achieved, to give the hoped-for pregnancy the best chance of success.

Travel

Travel plans should be made with caution if there is a possibility of pregnancy. The safest time to travel during pregnancy is in the middle trimester. Suggest that couples avoid long flights and travelling to areas where there is a risk of malaria.

Smoking cessation

This is likely to be the most common issue encountered [24,25]. Women who smoke should be informed that this may reduce their fertility[26]. Use a supportive and non-judgemental approach in order to boost the person's motivation and their sense of personal effectiveness. Many smokers say that they will stop when they conceive. This is an unwise strategy because they will not avoid the early pregnancy risks associated with smoking. They may also find smoking cessation more difficult than they anticipate and might need to use nicotine replacement or bupropion to help them stop, which are hazardous during pregnancy, though nicotine can be used if necessary. In addition, smoking has adverse nutritional effects and can lead to increased cadmium levels[27].

It is important for the woman's partner to stop smoking too, in order to provide her, and eventually the baby, with a smoke-free environment. There is also an association between smoking and reduced semen quality[28] (although the impact on male fertility is uncertain). If both partners smoke, giving up together provides increased motivation and support. Ideally, couples should stop smoking at least three months before conception. This and other addictions may require specialist help and advice.

Drugs

Women of childbearing age should be prioritised for drug dependency treatment, using an approach to minimise harm, possibly involving the use of methadone, buprenorphine or other substitution therapy[29]. Recreational drugs including cannabis, cocaine and amphetamines present serious hazards in pregnancy and should be avoided. Women dependent on opiates present a particular problem, as their babies are subject to a number of risks. Also, they may not be motivated to use contraception effectively or to cease their opiate use. Every effort should be made to discourage and help prevent pregnancy in opiate users until they overcome their addiction.

Record-keeping

It is good practice to record advice and treatment given, to support care of the individual and audit of treatment for the population as a whole. Records should be kept in an accessible, preferably electronic format, with appropriate coding of data.

Audit

Pre-conception care can be audited in terms of the number of people reached and the quality of care provided. This work could also support research on the outcomes of care.

Team work

Each primary care team will need to consider how best to deliver pre-conception care to its population and the roles of each team member. Possible roles include the following:

- **Midwife**: give advice to identified patients referred. Develop skills in preconception care for particular patient groups. Identify clients who have had a poor pregnancy outcome and who may require specific help in a future pregnancy and refer to physician.

- **Practice nurse**: use opportunistic contacts in new patient registration medicals, well-woman, contraception and smear clinics to give simple pre-conception advice and identify people planning a pregnancy. Ensure that women with chronic problems, including diabetes and epilepsy, who have childbearing potential are given opportunistic advice and educated about the need for preconception care. Refer people identified as being at risk of STIs. Offer chlamydia screening if available to appropriate cases.

- **Health visitor**: use routine contacts with families to give opportunistic advice to clients planning another pregnancy, and refer to physician when appropriate. Incorporate pregnancy preparation advice into regular health education activities.

- **Dietician**: develop dietary advice package tailored to preconception patients.

- **Doctors**: develop expertise in preconception care. It would perhaps be best for one partner to accept referrals for complex cases in this field. At present, few gynaecologists would be well placed to offer this service and it is best delivered in a primary care setting.

- **Secondary care**: referral to obstetricians, diabetologists, neurologists, genitourinary medicine, geneticists, rehabilitation physicians for specialist input when required. Similarly these professionals can use their contacts to identify women who may become pregnant and offer them advice and refer them back to the primary care team.

HOW TO CONTACT THE TARGET AUDIENCE

At primary care team level

Have a written policy for preconception care that includes the following:

- Opportunistic individual advice at registration, well woman clinic, contraception and cervical cytology appointments will enable the team to contact most of the target population. Computer templates used for recording data at these clinics can be made to include a prompt to discuss preconception care. Most people planning pregnancy do not announce this to their doctors at present in the UK, and many pregnancies are unplanned. Therefore the strategy should include advice targeted at all women. Other contacts will be generated by the team as detailed above.

- Include preconception care in the practice's chronic disease management protocols. If computer templates are used for diabetes and epilepsy, these can be made to include a prompt to consider pre-conception advice for women in the appropriate age group.

- Publicise the service in the waiting room and practice literature.

- After poor pregnancy outcomes, ensure that couples are offered preconception care sensitively at an appropriate time.

- Have available the book *Tommy's Guide to Pre-Pregnancy Care*[30].

Local action

- Work with local schools, young people's groups and women's groups to raise awareness of the benefits of pregnancy planning and preparation. This work can link with local action on teenage pregnancy and with Sure Start schemes, for example.

- Improve publicity locally for preconception care and education. Primary care organisations (PCOs – PCTs in England) to commission services from their local providers in a co-ordinated way across the locality.

- Local authorities and PCOs to support neighbourhood regeneration and community food projects.

National policy

- For those concerned about the risks of, and screening for, Down's Syndrome or Sickle Cell Disease when planning a pregnancy, the National Screening Committee runs an Antenatal and Newborn Screening Programme which co-ordinates screening for these conditions. The programme is to be expanded to include a wide range of other conditions such as congenital heart disease, hepatitis B and rubella.

- Steps need to be taken to improve nutrition for all children and young people, especially those on low incomes. This includes increasing benefit levels to enable families to purchase a good diet, increasing access to free school meals and the Welfare Foods Scheme, and health visiting input to couples before pregnancy[31].

- Government should make it the responsibility of PCOs to commission primary care or other services to provide preconception care to patients who need it, and publicise the availability of this.

- Fiscal and other measures such as advertising bans can reduce smoking in the population and these should be a greater priority in view of the effects on pregnancy.

FUTURE RESEARCH AND DEVELOPMENT

At present there is a limited evidence base for preconception care. It is a difficult topic to research with many practical and ethical obstacles. Priorities are to understand the decisions people make about planning and preparing for pregnancy, to evaluate interventions to improve outcomes, particularly smoking cessation and nutritional interventions, and to find the most effective modes of delivering services to people most at risk.

Key messages

- While there is a limited evidence base for preconception care, sufficient evidence is available to indicate that significant health improvements could result from a programme of preconception care.

- Areas to cover during history taking include the woman's or couple's reproductive history, their obstetric history, relationships history, smoking, alcohol and other drugs, environmental hazards, genetics, dietary history, chronic diseases and immunisation status.

- If there are risk factors that can be improved, such as smoking, obesity or other hazards, it may be wise to use a reversible contraceptive method until this is achieved.

- Each primary care team will need to consider the roles of each team member in delivering preconception care to its population.

- Any strategy for preconception care should include strategies for targeting all women. A written policy should highlight opportunities for discussing preconception care, for example, at registration, well woman clinic, contraception and cervical cytology appointments. The service should also be publicised in the waiting room and through practice literature.

References

1. Heyes T, Long S and Mathers N. Preconception care practice and beliefs of primary care workers. *Family Practitioner,* vol 21, no 1, 2004, pp22–27.

2. Spencer N. *Weighing the Evidence.* Abingdon: Radcliffe Medical Press 2003.

3. de Onis M, Villar J and Gulmezoglu M. Nutritional interventions to prevent intrauterine growth retardation: evidence from randomized controlled trials. *European Journal of Clinical Nutrition*, vol 52, suppl 1, 1998, pp83–93.

4. Merialdi M et al. Nutritional interventions during pregnancy for the prevention or treatment of impaired fetal growth: an overview of randomized controlled trials. *Journal of Nutrition*, vol 133, no 5, suppl 2, 2003, pp1626–1631.

5. Villar J, Gulmezoglu A, and de Onis M. Nutritional and antimicrobial interventions to prevent preterm birth: an overview of randomized controlled trials. *Obstetrical and Gynecological Survey*, vol 53, no 9, 1998, pp575–85.

6. Wald N and Hackshaw A. Folic acid and prevention of neural–tube defects. *Lancet*, vol 350, no 9078, 1997, p665.

7. de Weerd S et al. Preconception counseling improves folate status of women planning pregnancy. *Obstetrics and Gynecology*, vol 99, no 1, (2002) pp45–50.

8. Egen V and Hasford J. Prevention of neural tube defects: effect of an intervention aimed at implementing the official recommendations. *Sozial und Praventivmedizin*, vol 48, no 1, 2003, pp24–32.

9. See note 2 above.

10. Li D, Liu L, and Odouli R. Exposure to non-steroidal anti-inflammatory drugs during pregnancy and risk of miscarriage: population based cohort study. *British Medical Journal*, vol 327, no 7411, 2003, pp368–70.

11. Olsen, S and Secher N. A possible preventive effect of low-dose fish oil on early delivery and pre-eclampsia: indications from a 50-year-old controlled trial. *British Journal of Nutrition,* vol 64, no 3, 1990, pp599–609.

12. Rogers I and Emmett P. Avon Longitudinal Study of Pregnancy and Childhood. Diet during pregnancy in a population of pregnant women in South West England. *European Journal of Clinical Nutrition,* vol 52, no 4, 1998, pp246–50.

13. Food Standards Agency. *Fish in Pregnancy*. http://www.food.gov.uk 2003.

14. Food Standards Agency. *Eating in Pregnancy*. http://www.food.gov.uk 2003.

15. Ray J, O'Brien T and Chan W. Preconception care and the risk of congenital anomalies in the offspring of women with diabetes mellitus: a meta-analysis. *QJM*, vol 94, no 8, 2001, pp435–44.

16. Klinke J and Toth E L. Preconception care for women with type 1 diabetes. *Canadian Family Physician*, vol 49, no 6, 2003, pp769–73.

17. Oguni M et al. Improved pregnancy outcome in epileptic women in the last decade: relationship to maternal anticonvulsant therapy. *Brain and Development,* vol 14, no 6, 1992, pp371–80.

18. Custovic A et al. Effect of environmental manipulation in pregnancy and early life on respiratory symptoms and atopy during first year of life: a randomised trial. *Lancet*, vol 358, no 9277, 2001, pp188–93.

19. Wergeland E and Strand K. Work pace control and pregnancy health in a population-based sample of employed women in Norway. *Scandinavian Journal of Work and Environment Health*, vol 24, no 3, 1998, pp206–12.

20. Li D et al. A population-based prospective cohort study of personal exposure to magnetic fields during pregnancy and the risk of miscarriage. *Epidemiology*, vol 13, no 1, 2002, pp9–20.

21. Toppenberg K, Hill D and Miller D. Safety of radiographic imaging during pregnancy. *American Family Physician*, vol 59, no 7, 1999, pp1813–18,1820.

22. Department of Health. Dental Amalgam. http://www.dh.gov.uk 2003.

23. National Institute for Clinical Excellence (NICE). *Fertility: Assessment and Treatment for People with Fertility Problems*. NICE 2004.

24. de Weerd S et al. Maternal smoking cessation intervention: targeting women and their partners before pregnancy. *American Journal of Public Health*, vol 91, no 11, 2001, pp 1733–34.

25. Hruba D and Kachlik P. Influence of maternal active and passive smoking during pregnancy on birthweight in newborns. *Central European Journal of Public Health*, vol 8, no 4, 2000, pp249–52.

26. See note 23 above.

27. Shiverick K and Salafia C. Cigarette smoking and pregnancy I: ovarian, uterine and placental effects. *Placenta*, vol 20, no 4, 1999, pp265–272.

28. British Medical Association (BMA) Board of Science and Education and Tobacco Control Resource Centre. *The Impact of Smoking on Sexual, Reproductive and Child Health*. London: BMA 2004. Available at http://www.bma.org.uk/ap.nsf/Content/SmokingReproductiveLife

29. Schindler S et al. Neonatal outcome following buprenorphine maintenance during conception and throughout pregnancy, *Addiction*, vol 98, no 1, 2003, pp 103–10.

30. Tassoni, P. *Tommy's Guide to Pre-pregnancy Care.* London: Tommy's (the baby charity) 2003.

31. The Maternity Alliance. *Report of the Preconception Care Conference and Follow Up Meeting*. Maternity Alliance 2002. Available at http://www.maternityalliance.org.uk

Links to evidence-based guidelines and policies

Key texts

Tassoni P. *Tommy's Guide to Pre-Pregnancy Care*. London: Tommy's (The baby charity) 2003.

Spencer N. *Weighing the Evidence: How is birthweight determined?* Radcliffe Medical Press 2003.

Cefalo R and Moos M-K. *Preconceptional Health Care: A practical guide*. USA: Mosby-Year Book 1995.

Prodigy guidelines – see www.prodigy.nhs.uk

Useful websites

www.prodigy.nhs.uk
Authoritative guidance on pre-conceptual care in a range of situations.

www.nelh.nhs.uk
Information from the National Electronic Library for Health on screening programmes in the antenatal and newborn periods.

www.nsc.nhs.uk
National Screening Committee website.

www.toxnet.nlm.nih.gov
Free access US toxicology database site.

www.spib.axl.co.uk
Toxicology database for NHS departments and GPs only – password needed.

www.foodstandards.gov.uk
Excellent summary of dietary and food safety advice.

www.tommys-campaign.org
UK charity with the aim of preventing premature birth, miscarriage and stillbirth.

http://health.yahoo.com/health/centers/pregnancy/202.html
Advice about fertility and conception.

http://archive.food.gov.uk/dept_health/pdf/amalgam.pdf
Information about dental amalgam and health.

www.maternityalliance.org.uk
Information and campaigns to support pregnancy, particularly benefits and rights.

www.miscarriageassociation.org.uk
Help for women and their families.

www.rcog.org.uk
Guidance and information for women, and health professionals, on haemolytic streptococcus Group B.

Useful organisations

NHS Smoking Helpline
0800 169 0 169

Quit Smoking Helpline
0800 00 22 00

NHS Pregnancy Smoking Helpline
0800 169 9 169

Chapter 5

ABORTION

Kate Guthrie

INTRODUCTION

This chapter looks at the delivery of abortion services from a primary care perspective. It begins with an overview of abortion services within the UK and discusses how women access services. Different abortion procedures, and possible complications, are considered. The chapter then focuses on follow-up in primary care and what needs to be in place to ensure that services are quick, efficient and caring. The final summary draws together the key points of the chapter.

OVERVIEW

Legally, women in Scotland, England and Wales achieved the right to request the termination of an unwanted pregnancy with the 1967 Abortion Act, which was then amended in 1990 (see Box 5.1, page 138). The Act does not apply in Northern Ireland or the Isle of Man (see Annex 1, page 152 for further details).

While the 1967 Abortion Act has given women the right to request an abortion, this right needs to be matched with a service that is also accessible, appropriate, and of high standard across primary, secondary and tertiary care.

The NHS Plan and the National Sexual Health Strategies have made local doctors and nurses in primary care trusts responsible for shaping and commissioning abortion services to ensure that they are modern, patient-friendly and of sufficiently high quality. As the NHS access point of care, primary care staff therefore play a key role in the delivery of abortion services.

A key target within the strategies is to address the disparities that exist within abortion services across the country. The introduction of specialist GP services, complemented by family planning/sexual health services, gives the opportunity for putting the patient at the centre, ending the current postcode lottery of service provision. For this to happen, effective commissioning is required using the service network and care pathway approach. All this needs to be underpinned by robust clinical governance arrangements. The Recommended Standards for Sexual Health Services, published in 2005, clearly lay down principles of care for abortion provision and provide a framework for service design and delivery.

Box 5.1:

Statutory grounds for termination of pregnancy

(based on the Abortion Act 1967 with amendments made in the Human Fertilisation and Embryology Act 1990)

A legally induced abortion must be certified by two registered medical practitioners as justified under one or more of the following grounds:

A the continuance of the pregnancy would involve risk to the life of the pregnant woman greater than if the pregnancy were terminated

B the termination is necessary to prevent grave permanent injury to the physical or mental health of the pregnant woman

C the pregnancy has **not** exceeded its 24th week and that the continuance of the pregnancy would involve risk, greater than if the pregnancy were terminated, of injury to the physical or mental health of the pregnant woman

D the pregnancy has **not** exceeded its 24th week and that the continuance of the pregnancy would involve risk, greater than if the pregnancy were terminated, of injury to the physical or mental health of the existing child(ren) of the family of the pregnant woman

E there is a substantial risk that if the child were born it would suffer from such physical or mental abnormalities as to be seriously handicapped.

The regulations also permit abortion to be performed in an emergency on the basis of the signature of the doctor performing the procedure – which may be provided up to 24 hours after the termination. The emergency grounds are:

F to save the life of the pregnant woman

G to prevent grave permanent injury to the physical or mental health of the pregnant woman.

ACCESS

Women have to know that a service exists and how to access it early and easily if they are to be given safe choices of abortion methods. Level 1 of the National Strategy for Sexual Health and HIV includes pregnancy testing and states that referral should be available in every general practice[1,2]. For this, women need clear, accessible signposting. A multimedia approach is needed to cover all patient groups.

Information on local access to abortion should be available via websites, posters in surgeries, clubs and leisure venues, and listings in the White and Yellow Pages of telephone and web directories. Local radio advertisements and widely promoted telephone helplines are also effective.

Signposting to other related services within primary care, such as family planning and sexual health clinics, is also important. Emergency access should be possible either as a walk-in or triage service. For this, there should be robust standards for clerical and reception staff to follow so a woman can request and receive an urgent appointment in confidence. A useful system is a card which can be picked up and shown to the receptionist when confidential, emergency sexual health care is needed – for example, emergency contraception, urgent pregnancy testing or pregnancy counselling. Hence, the receptionist knows the nature of the request without the need for the woman to discuss this in the public reception area, and she can therefore arrange an urgent consultation.

In order to maintain confidentiality, all discussions with the woman should take place in a private environment. No assumptions should be made about the woman or her reasons for accessing abortion. It may be that things have happened to her that she has chosen not to disclose at this stage.

Ensuring speedy access to services

A woman should be able to access free and confidential pregnancy testing at clearly advertised locations which need not be clinical, for example, youth advisory services, but should include primary care. Ideally, this would be an on-the-spot confirmatory pregnancy test and a pharmacist/clinician should supply initial written and verbal information on the choices available locally to someone with an unplanned pregnancy, including abortion, adoption and motherhood. This consultation must give accurate and unbiased information and non-directive support to enable informed choice. It can be explained to women who have done 'home pregnancy tests' that the results, where positive, are usually correct, so there is no need for the clinician to repeat the test unless the woman is unsure.

It is important that the clinician assesses gestation by history and abdominal palpitation. If the pregnancy is of unknown or advanced gestation, accurate dating will be needed to inform the woman of what choices she has, and to speed up access to abortion services, if that is what she elects. This initial brief clinical examination can be confirmed later by a more thorough clinical examination, or preferably by scan.

To maximise accessibility to abortion services onward referral should be speedy: direct access by the woman is the ideal, otherwise referral via a telephone helpline, fax, email or first class post to a 'safe haven' and certainly within five days of first contact with the healthcare profession[3]. The later the procedure the greater the risk of complications and potentially, the more limited the choice of procedures locally. Moreover, abortions over 24 weeks' gestation are not available under clauses C and D of the Act. (In 2003, less than 1 per cent of legal abortions that took place were 22 weeks and over[4].) If, for ethical or religious reasons the clinician cannot support a request for abortion referral, they have a duty to promptly refer to someone who can supply the necessary information services.

Box 5.2:

Good professional practice

Doctors providing abortion care are bound by the same *duties of a doctor* as laid down by the GMC as for all other aspects of their clinical practice. The United Kingdom Central Council for Nursing, Midwifery and Health Visiting (UKCC) (now the Nursing & Midwifery Council, NMC) published a Code of Professional Conduct and Guidelines for Professional Practice equivalent to the GMC's *Duties of a Doctor*:

- Make the care of your patient your first concern.
- Treat every patient politely and considerately.
- Respect patients' dignity and privacy.
- Listen to patients and respect their views.
- Give patients information in a way they can understand.
- Respect the right of patients to be fully involved in decisions about their care.
- Keep your professional knowledge and skills up-to-date.
- Recognise the limits of your professional competence.
- Be honest and trustworthy.
- Respect and protect confidential information.
- Make sure that your personal beliefs do not prejudice your patients' care.
- Act quickly to protect patients from risk if you have good reason to believe that you or a colleague may not be fit to practice.
- Avoid abusing your position as a doctor.
- Work with colleagues in the ways that best serve patients' interests.

Making services accessible to young women

The practice or clinic should have strategies in place to ensure that their services are accessible to young people. A young person's age is not a bar to confidentiality

or services. As with contraception, a young woman under the age of 16 can consent
to an abortion without parental consent or knowledge if the clinician believes
that she exhibits the capacity to consent by fulfilling 'Fraser criteria' (see Box 5.3,
below). The document *Protecting the Public: Strengthening Protection Against
Sex Offenders and Reforming the Law on Sexual Offences*[5] does not alter this. The
exception is those young women who are wards of court who require the court's
agreement for abortion to proceed.

Box 5.3:

Fraser criteria to assess capacity to consent (see also Department of Health guidance for
health professionals on treating under-16s[6])

The doctor is justified in proceeding without the parent's consent or knowledge if:

- the girl (under 16) understands their advice
- they cannot persuade her to inform her parents or allow them to inform the parents that she
  is seeking contraceptive advice
- she is likely to continue having sexual intercourse with, or without contraceptive advice
- unless she receives contraceptive advice or treatment her physical or mental health, or
  both, are likely to suffer
- her best interests require them to give her contraceptive advice, treatment or both, without
  parental consent.

If there is any case of doubt about the young woman's competence to consent,
then the clinician should discuss the case with a more senior doctor, usually the
consultant running the abortion services (Level 3 provider) who in turn should
make ready recourse to legal advice. Furthermore, all staff must also be alert to
the possibilities of child abuse and non-consensual sexual activity, especially if
a young or vulnerable person refuses to involve her family, is accompanied by a
controlling adult or is acting inappropriately for her age. If abuse is suspected, as the
interest of the young person (and any siblings or other vulnerable young person)
is paramount, the doctor is required to disclose information to the appropriate
statutory service as laid down in local child protection guidelines. If this includes
breaking confidentiality, the young person must be informed why (provided this
does not compromise her safety or the safety of other young people) and offered all
necessary help and support.

Box 5.4:

Special protection for children and the most vulnerable

(From *Protecting the Public: Strengthening Protection Against Sex Offenders and Reforming the Law on Sexual Offences*, Chapter 4, 2004)

There may be circumstances where sexual activity takes place with the apparent consent of both parties but where one of the parties is in such a position of power over the other that the sexual activity is wrong and should come within the realms of criminal law. These circumstances include:

- adult sexual activity with a child
- sexual activity between minors
- sexual grooming
- familial sexual abuse of a child
- prohibited adult sexual relationships
- abuse of position of trust
- sexual activity with a person who did not, by reason of a learning disability or mental disorder at that time, have the capacity to consent
- obtaining sexual activity by inducement, threat or deception with a person who has a learning disability or mental disorder
- breach of a relationship of care.

Making services accessible to other groups of women

The practice or clinic should also have strategies in place to support other groups who traditionally find access difficult. This includes women from ethnic minorities (for example, access to translators or counsellors aware of religious or cultural requirements), and those who are disabled (for example, British Sign Language interpreters).

REFERRING WITHOUT DELAY

If abortion is potentially the woman's way of dealing with an unplanned pregnancy, but she is still unsure, she should be referred into the abortion service without delay. However, it is important to stress to the woman that she is not obliged to undergo the abortion, and that this is a way of ensuring that no time is lost, should this be her chosen path. Being seen by a clinician can be deferred to provide the opportunity for counselling and further support in decision-making, as well as access to social services if required, but at least she is within the service so arrangements to provide an abortion can be made speedily, if this is her final decision. It is also helpful if the primary carer is able to sign the certificate HSA1 giving legal support to the abortion request. If not, this should be completed by the providers of the abortion service itself.

If possible, the issues of counselling, contraception and sexual health screening should be raised at an early stage, ideally by the person the woman presents to for help with her unplanned pregnancy. These issues can be arranged in primary care but if not, they should certainly be picked up by abortion service providers. All are aspects of a holistic abortion service and should be part of the service protocol. Women undergoing abortion are a high-risk group for sexually transmissible infections (STIs), hence screening and routine antibiotic prophylaxis is recommended. Raising these issues early on can lead to partner notification and address the public health aspect of infection[7].

In 2003, about 30 per cent of women undergoing abortion in England and Wales had undergone one or more previous abortions[8].

If contraception is discussed with the woman at an early stage in the process, the chosen method can be initiated immediately post-procedure – ovulation is within a month of first trimester abortion in over 90 per cent of women[9]. There is also the potential for fitting an IUD/IUS or implant at the time of abortion. Sterilisation can also be performed at the time of surgery if the woman was awaiting sterilisation anyway. However, the Royal College guidelines[10] on sterilisation stress the increased failure rate of such sterilising procedures and the element of regret. Women may understandably find it difficult to make decisions about long-term contraception while stressed due to the current unplanned pregnancy. Regretting expensive but reversible methods of contraception is financially wasteful but remediable; regretting sterilisation is not. In reality, it has to be accepted that many women find it difficult to think about contraception at this stage in the process.

ABORTION PROCEDURES

Primary carers need to be able to give accurate verbal and written information to women about their local abortion providers and the methods of abortion available at different gestation bands. Ideally, the woman should have a choice of method of abortion. Information is therefore also needed about the advantages, disadvantages and risks of the various methods so that she can make an informed choice.

Having written information means that the woman can take it away with her and study it before the procedure. Leaflets are available from the Royal College of Obstetricians and Gynaecologists (www.rcog.org.uk) and **fpa** (www.fpa.org.uk). Local leaflets can be adapted from these, adding in local information from audit, such as complication rates. These should be available in different languages and media, for example, audiotape. Women who do not speak English have been found to have an increased incidence of not being able to read in their own language.

Information should also be available on associated services (contraception, genitourinary medicine, counselling) and for partners and carers.

Box 5.5:

Recommended methods of abortion (RCOG 2004[11])
Recommended methods of abortion for different gestations (weeks from last menstrual period, regular 28-day cycle):

- up to 7 weeks: aspiration under strict protocol (to reduce the risk of failing to terminate)
- diagnosis to 59 days post-conception: medical abortion using mifepristone and prostaglandin
- 7–15 weeks: suction termination (sharp curettage not employed)
- 9–24 weeks: medical abortion using mifepristone and multiple doses of prostaglandin
- 15–24 weeks: surgical abortion by dilatation and evacuation. Feticide is required after 21 weeks.

It may be that the local commissioners have outsourced the service from an independent sector provider. They should provide all the above equally as effectively as an NHS provider.

Box 5.6:

Percentage of abortions performed by NHS Agencies in 2002

Gestation (weeks)	Total number	% NHS agency
0–12	153,730	33.5
13–14	9,573	50.2
15–16	5,491	59.7
17–19	4,246	63.4
20–21	1,512	61.8
22–23	1,245	63.3

Department of Health. Abortion statistics, England and Wales: 2002. Department of Health, July 2004. Bulletin 2002/23, revised edition.

Services should be available for all gestation bands and unrestricted by age, gestation, income, parity or marital status and a choice should be available at all gestations. Waiting times from referral to procedure should not exceed a maximum of three weeks and women should be cared for separately from other gynaecology patients[12].

Surgical abortions can be performed under local anaesthetic, conscious sedation or general anaesthetic. In the UK, local anaesthetic is not often used above ten weeks' gestation. Most abortions under 20 weeks' gestation can be performed as day cases provided women have no significant medical conditions and they can be discharged home to carers with ready access to medical care.

Medical abortion regimes in the UK use the progesterone antagonist, Mifepristone, followed at 36/48 hours later by a prostaglandin analogue. Both drugs have to be taken within their licensed unit to comply with legislation. Up to 13 weeks' gestation, 95 per cent of abortions are complete on the day of the procedure and the vast majority are performed as outpatients. At 13–21 weeks, 66 per cent are day cases and 9 per cent require uterine evacuation due to a retained placenta.

Patient acceptability studies have shown that provided women can choose the method of abortion, they are happy with their choice. Informed choice appears to be more important than the incidence of side effects in predicting acceptability. The British Pregnancy Advisory Service has studied women who have left the clinic one hour after prostaglandin administration (that is, they did not wait within the unit to abort). Seventy-six per cent reported that they would advise others to follow the rapid discharge protocol (personal communication). An **fpa** inspired UK survey of women undergoing medical abortion asked if they would have liked to take the prostaglandin analogue at home[13]. Only 36 per cent said that they would wish to do so. This indicates again that the important factor for women is having the choice.

An **fpa** study in 2002[14] also reported that women valued privacy and anonymity, a positive staff attitude and a service that eliminates delay but allows them the time, information and support to come to the right decision. Continuity of people and place was also important.

COMPLICATIONS OF ABORTION

Once pregnant, a woman only has two choices: continuing the pregnancy to term or having an abortion. Both can have complications. Unfortunately, hoping that the pregnancy will miscarry or being in denial of the pregnancy are two reasons why (particularly young) women present late to abortion services. Statistically, abortion is the safer of the two options. A woman needs to know what the potential complications of both choices are to make an informed decision as to whether to continue the pregnancy or not, as embodied in the NHS 'consent to treatment' form.

When considering an abortion, a woman must be made aware of:

- what the possible complications are

- their incidence locally (preferably from local audit, or from national figures)

- how to identify if one of these complications is happening to her

- who to contact for help. Ideally, this should be in the form of a 24-hour telephone helpline.

This should be given both verbally and in writing, as part of pre-procedure information-giving. It could be included in a pre-printed consent form, a copy of which the woman retains[15].

Box 5.7:

Information required by women requesting abortion (RCOG 2004[16])

Professionals involved in abortion care should be equipped to provide women with accurate information relating to the following topics:

- that abortion is safer than continuing a pregnancy to term and that complications are uncommon

- description of the method(s) of abortion available within the local service for particular gestations

- immediate complications including: haemorrhage, uterine perforation, cervical lacerations, and anaesthetic complications. Women must be informed that should one of these complications occur, further treatment in the form of blood transfusion, laparoscopy or laparotomy may be required

- complications in the early weeks following abortion including: incomplete abortion requiring re-evacuation, continuing pregnancy requiring a further abortion procedure, pelvic infection, and short-term emotional distress

- long-term effects, which may, rarely, be associated with abortion including: miscarriage or preterm birth and psychological problems

- conditions where an association with abortion has been postulated but where evidence provides reassurance (for example, breast cancer, infertility).

Immediate complications

These will occur at the time of the abortion procedure. They are uncommon, and mainly associated with surgical methods of abortion (see Box 5.7 above). All increase with an advance in gestation and reduction in clinician experience. Pre-existing maternal factors must also be taken into account, such as a history of repeated/complications of caesarean section, or haemorrhagic disorder.

Complications in the early weeks post-procedure

These complications can be identified by the patient if she knows what to look for, but may be ignored due to denial, shame or incomplete understanding, or inadequate information-giving (see Box 5.7, page 146). Unfortunately, services find that despite giving follow-up appointments routinely or selectively, non-attendance rates are high, so often women have no routine clinical supervision. Consequently, any service structure should provide a system of open and rapid access for review should the need arise. In reality, many women turn to their primary carer for help.

Infection, retained products and a missed ectopic pregnancy will present with bleeding and/or lower abdominal pain although in the initial phases all could be silent. Pelvic infection can also be associated with vaginal discharge, pyrexia or simply a feeling of 'just not being well' with no other specific features. It can also coexist with retained products. Investigations include triple swabs and pelvic ultrasound, with empirical antibiotic prescribing if infection is suspected to reduce the chance of tubal disease.

In the UK, the incidence of post-abortal infection has been reduced by pre-procedure screening and treatment of infection, routine antibiotic prophylaxis and active management of retained products (whether the management is medical, surgical or expectant).

Both an ongoing pregnancy and an ectopic pregnancy may present with an absence of a normal next period and continuing symptoms of pregnancy. It should be suspected if a surgical abortion was performed at a gestation of six weeks or less or in the presence of a uterine abnormality. Pregnancy will be confirmed by serum BhCG and ultrasound. The failure rate of early medical and surgical abortion has been quoted as around 0.9 and 0.5 per cent respectively, the former being dependent on the drug regime.

Short-term emotional distress is common after abortion. It should be anticipated and dealt with sympathetically and non-judgementally. This can be associated with lack of knowledge/fantasies which the woman did not want to address pre-operatively, for example, 'Did the fetus feel pain?', 'What did it look like?'. Tackling these questions honestly usually resolves unfounded fears and grief.

Long-term effects

Women's greatest expressed fear is of subfertility. There is no increased risk of this provided the abortion itself was uncomplicated by infection or injury.

An increased risk of placenta praevia in future pregnancies appears to exist in association with sharp curettage (as opposed to the now commonly used aspiration curettage) as the method of surgical abortion. There is limited evidence as to whether there is or is not an increased incidence of miscarriage or preterm birth.

The current evidence is that there is no increased incidence of breast cancer.

Long-term psychological repercussions of abortion are a contested topic which are deserving of further research. Certain groups of women have been identified as being at increased risk of psychological morbidity[17] (for example, pre-procedure ambivalence, lack of supportive partner, a psychiatric history, membership of a cultural group that considers abortion wrong). They should be identified if possible, and the circumstances acknowledged and managed proactively as part of pre-procedure care. The most recent evidence from Europe is that abortion per se carries increased psychological risk. Although there are confounding factors in interpreting this data, it must be accepted as it currently stands and awareness be raised. If a pro-choice stance is to be taken by the clinician, it is incumbent upon her or him to ensure that the patient is aware of the tensions between resolving immediate problems and the potential of long-term regret and guilt. This can be difficult when working within a limited time frame with a distressed woman whose immediate problems cloud her ability to see the future. This is where rapid access to specialist counsellors is essential for decision-making and post-procedure support, whatever decision the woman arrives at.

FOLLOW-UP IN PRIMARY CARE

If the woman can see her primary carer about two weeks after the procedure, her physical and psychological state can be assessed. She only need be physically examined if she:

- has significant persistent vaginal loss (reducing loss is to be expected with medical procedures, and may also be affected by the method of contraception, for example, progestogen-only contraceptives)
- has symptoms of infection (generalised lower abdominal pain, pyrexia, offensive discharge, dyspareunia, 'just not feeling well')
- requires to have the presence of intrauterine contraception checked.

The woman's psychological wellbeing needs to be sensitively explored. This includes reassuring her that she can come back for help if she feels that any aspect of her wellbeing has become affected by the experience, or she thinks that she is developing a complication. This visit is an opportunity to review contraception again and to provide any ongoing supplies, including condoms, for the prevention of infection if appropriate. If she has undergone a medical abortion under 63 days or a surgical procedure under seven weeks, the normality of the next period must be emphasised as confirmation of a complete procedure. If in doubt, a screening BhCG should be sought.

Most importantly, the follow-up in primary care is an opportunity for the woman to see her primary carer as a non-judgemental person she can turn to in a crisis and who will be there to help support her through it, with the door left open for whatever the future holds.

SERVICE ORGANISATION

Abortion services are core to the implementation of the National Sexual Health Strategy of Scotland, England and Wales. They are part of service organisation at Level 3 of the strategy (specialist providers and commissioners) which spans primary, secondary and tertiary care. Ideally, this requires the commissioning of an organised network of services underpinned by a care pathway. Ideally, if the pathway is truly patient-centred, this begins when the woman suspects she may be pregnant, but in reality it usually starts at first patient contact (usually in primary care although not so in direct access services) and ends at follow-up from the procedure or exiting from care. By definition, this is supported by evidence-based guidelines and specialist policies for the management of special-needs groups, specifically young people. The evidence to date is that services *can* be quick, efficient and caring if championed and managed effectively. This includes:

- **Confidentiality**: there is patient fear of condemnation and prejudice, which is not unfounded in society today.

- **Easy access**: this requires the advertising of services (preferably direct access) and service providers, with non-directive onward referral from primary carers who feel that they themselves cannot provide the service. Women need to know who they can turn to in a crisis and have the right to expect a responsive service centred on their declared needs. Flow into each subsequent stage or branch of the pathway should be speedy but not rushed.

- **Adherence to standards**: the Faculty of Family Planning, **fpa** and the RCOG have published these among others. The recommended standards and networks for sexual health services[18], commissioned by the Department of Health, were published in March 2005, and provide clear standards, interventions, audit indicators and implications for service planning for the many services that make a fully comprehensive abortion service. These include service access, pregnancy testing, abortion service provision and sexual health service networks.

- **A trained workforce of adequate size and resource to offer a prompt and comprehensive service**: a challenge to service provision is the decreasing numbers of surgeons willing to be trained in the skills of abortion procedures, particularly beyond 15 weeks – dilatation, evacuation and late surgical procedures. If insufficient surgeons are available then this will cease to be an option available to women as an abortion method. (The Faculty of Family Planning is developing a training programme to address this service issue so that women can continue to have the choice and, hence, attain service satisfaction at a traumatic time in their lives.) A survey in Newcastle has shown that despite thorough counselling about the reduced risks of medical versus late surgical abortion, 75 per cent of women still opted for the surgical procedure, mainly due to a desire to be unaware during the procedure. It is clear that in the future, nurses will play an increasing role in abortion provision.

- **Patient information**: without information given in a manner understandable to any given individual and their partners/carers of what, where, why, who and when, there cannot be true informed choice and consent.

- **User/carer representation in service design and delivery**: this is essential to ensure that all of the above is appropriate for the population served, and to address issues which cannot be second-guessed by service providers as they traditionally have been in the past.

SUMMARY

What to do about an unplanned pregnancy is one of the biggest and hardest decisions a woman will ever have to make. By UK law, she has the right to be considered for abortion of that pregnancy (along with limited grounds in Northern Ireland).

Therapeutic abortion is a safe procedure provided that high standards of clinical care are followed, as laid down in nationally available clinical guidelines. Currently, in Scotland, England and Wales, service availability is very variable, and not standardised. As gatekeepers to services, and as laid down in the National Sexual Health Strategies, primary carers have a crucial role to play in information-giving and enabling access to services at Level 1. They are also able to provide some specialist services at Level 2. Their attitude and care for the woman will significantly colour her views about her abortion, and can turn what may be potentially a miserable and judgemental experience into a positive one from which she can grow and move on with her life.

Key messages

- Adequate abortion provision is a key target in the National Sexual Health Strategy.
- There are evidence based clinical guidelines upon which services can be based (RCOG[19]).
- Accessibility to free and rapid pregnancy testing and rapid referral (preferably self-referral) to abortion services is key to reducing the gestation at abortion, desired as safer, less psychologically traumatic and enables choice of method.
- The recommended standards for sexual health services[20] are for all settings providing sexual health care, and service users, and are a valuable tool for planning service delivery in collaboration with service users.
- Abortion care should be a comprehensive package of care including sexual health screening, contraception provision and social and emotional support, geared to enable women to make informed choices based on high quality and understandable information.

Annex 1

THE LAW ON ABORTION IN NORTHERN IRELAND

The Abortion Act does not apply in Northern Ireland. Following a Judicial Review process, the law on abortion in Northern Ireland has been clarified for the first time and now states:

Abortion is legal in Northern Ireland when:

- the continuance of the pregnancy threatens the life of the mother, or would adversely affect her mental or physical health

- the adverse effect on her mental or physical health is a 'real and serious' one and permanent or long term

- the risk of the adverse effect occurring is a probability but a possibility can be regarded as sufficient if the imminent death of the mother was potentially the adverse effect.

In June 2001, **fpa** won the right to the first Judicial Review of medical practice relating to abortion and the provision of abortion services in Northern Ireland. The Review took place in March 2002 and in July 2002 Mr Justice Kerr concluded that the Department of Health, Social Services and Public Safety (DHSSPS) was not failing in its statutory duty to issue guidelines, but he thought it prudent if they did. **fpa** immediately lodged an appeal and in October 2004 Belfast High Court of Appeal ruled that the DHSSPS had failed to perform its statutory duties. In response to this, in 2005 the DHSSPS instigated a formal investigation into the provision of abortion services in Northern Ireland, which is ongoing[21].

THE LAW ON ABORTION IN THE ISLE OF MAN

The Isle of Man has its own Termination of Pregnancy (Medical Defences) Act 1995. While similar to the 1967 Abortion Act, the wording differs within the Isle of Man Act so that in reality, very few abortions take place. For example, Section 2 (1) b reads 'grave permanent injury . . .'. Many doctors would find it difficult to warrant that injury to the physical or mental health of the woman is permanent especially where mental health is concerned.

In cases where mental health is at risk, one of the doctors assessing the woman needs to be a consultant psychiatrist.

Section 5 of the Act looks at sexual crime. Here, the woman has to 'prove' that she has been raped or assaulted by producing written evidence or having to report the alleged assault or rape to the police. This includes incestuous sexual crime.

References

1. Medical Foundation for AIDS and Sexual Health. *The Recommended Standards for Sexual Health Services*. Medfash, 2005.

2. Department of Health. *The National Strategy for Sexual Health and HIV.* Department of Health 2001.

3. See note 1 above.

4. Department of Health, Abortion Statistics, England and Wales: Department of Health, July 2005, Bulletin 2004/14, revised edition.

5. *Protecting the Public: Strengthening Protection Against Sex Offenders and Reforming the Law on Sexual Offences.* Presented to Parliament November 2002. HMSO ID 111491 11/02 065536.

6. *Best Practice Guidance for Doctors and other Health Professionals on the Provision of Advice and Treatment to Young People under 16 on Contraception, Sexual and Reproductive Health*. Department of Health 2004.

7. Evidence-based Clinical Guideline no 7: *The Care of Women Requesting Induced Abortion.* Royal College of Obstetricians and Gynaecologists (RCOG) 2004. Available at http://www.rcog.org.uk

8. See note 4 above.

9. Cameron I and Baird D. The return to ovulation following early abortion: a comparison between vacuum aspiration and prostaglandin. *Endocrinologica,* vol 118, 1988, pp161–67.

10. *Evidence-based Clinical Guideline no 4. Male and Female Sterilisation.* RCOG 2004. Available at http://www.rcog.org.uk

11. See note 7 above.

12. *Effective Commissioning of Sexual Health and HIV Services. A sexual health and HIV commissioning toolkit for primary care trusts and local authorities.* January 2003. Available at http://www.doh.gov.uk/sexualhealthandhiv

13. Hamoda H, Critchley H, Paterson K et al. The acceptability of home medical abortion to women in UK settings. *British Journal of Obstetrics and Gynaecology,* 112 (6), 2005, pp781–5.

14. Mawer C and McGovern M. *Early Abortions: Promoting real choice for women.* **fpa** November 2003.

15. Guthrie K, Waudby C and Arnott P. Termination of pregnancy care pathway. Worth the effort? presented at the 8th Congress of the European Society of Contraception, Edinburgh June 2004.

16. See note 7 above.

17. See note 4 above.

18. See note 1 above.

19. See note 7 above.

20. See note 1 above.

21. **fpa**. *Abortion Factsheet*. **fpa** September 2005.

Chapter 6

SEXUALLY TRANSMISSIBLE INFECTIONS: A PRIMARY CARE PERSPECTIVE

Philippa Matthews and Helen Macaulay

INTRODUCTION

Rates of sexually transmissible infections (STIs) in the UK are rising out of control[1,2]. The consequences to health of STIs are significant [3,4]. Against this background, the role of the GP and practice nurse (PN) in detecting and managing STIs is becoming increasingly important. There is good evidence that primary care attenders have significant rates of sexually transmissible infection [5,6].

This chapter aims to support GPs and practice nurses who wish to respond to the certainty that many of their patients have STIs. Many of these patients may be unaware of this, and some will present in primary care. The chapter highlights key issues in the diagnosis and management of STIs in the general practice setting, focusing on issues which are not usually addressed by other sources on the subject.

Two or three decades ago the symptoms of STIs were considered to be quite narrow in range. Syphilis was rare and symptoms of other STIs generally related to the genitals: ulcers, warts, pubic lice and discharge. It was comparatively easy for the GP (and indeed the patient) to see that genitourinary medicine (GUM) attendance was appropriate. Unfortunately the clinical picture in primary care is now entirely different and much more complex. The symptoms of STIs are now recognised to be diverse, and may not affect the genitals. Symptoms can be short-lived or subtle. They may occur months or years after the infection was acquired. HIV can present to the GP with an enormous range of clinical conditions, many of which are commonplace in *non* HIV-infected patients (see Chapter 7). In women, chlamydia can mimic cystitis or cause menstrual disorders without any associated vaginal discharge. It can cause conjunctivitis in adults and neonates. The GP cannot simply refer all patients to the GUM clinic with, for example, intermenstrual bleeding or hard-to-treat seborrhoeic dermatitis. Yet the standard clinical training for primary care has, in most instances, failed to respond to this altered clinical picture and equip GPs with the clinical knowledge and skills that they require. Some of the more common (or more unusual) symptoms and signs of STIs are summarised in Table 6.2 for quick reference (see page 174).

In addition, all STIs – even those that may be causing serious harm – can be asymptomatic. Chlamydia can cause pelvic inflammation and tubal damage without any symptoms at all. HIV might be destroying a patient's T Lymphocytes until ultimately their immunity is significantly compromised and (for some) it is only then that the first symptoms occur. What can we do about asymptomatic STIs in primary care? At the very least, an awareness of the possibility of asymptomatic infection is important in a range of clinical circumstances, for instance, if we plan to fit an IUD, or if we prescribe oral contraception for a patient who had been using condoms as contraception. Risk assessment (see Chapter 2 on sexual history-taking) will help us to decide, with our patients, which tests are appropriate. Again, it is rarely practicable to ask all patients in such circumstances to attend GUM.

Specialist services provided for STI diagnosis and management in the UK are overwhelmed[7]. New strategies in primary care might enable GUM services to see, as a priority, patients for whom their expertise is most required, with the care of others being devolved. To date, little has been done to explore ways in which primary care could be supported to play its part in STI diagnosis and management. The 2004 contract for GPs in the UK may change this[8] by providing financial support for a minority of practices which opt in to STI care ('enhanced' services). The consequences of this for the patients of all the *other* practices are unclear. There may be a detrimental effect if such practices see it as unfunded work that they should drop (or continue to ignore) – perhaps maintaining the 'invisibility' of STIs in the primary care context.

There is currently little available information relevant to primary care on protocols, audit standards and computer templates for STI diagnosis and management. This is discussed on page 176.

There is excellent further information available on the epidemiology, physical consequences and management of each STI (and indeed other genital infections). Useful sources are listed in detail at the end of the chapter (see pages 179 to 181). They include regularly updated epidemiological information, detailed clinical information and photographs, and national management guidelines.

THE HANDBOOK OF SEXUAL HEALTH IN PRIMARY CARE

There are a number of steps which must be taken if an STI is to be correctly diagnosed and managed. These include:

- knowing which infections are transmissible sexually, and which are not
- being able to recognise that an STI may be present
- knowing the important clinical consequences of individual STIs – treated or untreated
- being able to confirm the diagnosis
- knowing which other STIs need to be tested for, once an STI diagnosis is confirmed
- knowing what treatment is required
- knowing what information the patient will need
- knowing when partner notification is (and is not) required
- knowing when a test of cure may be helpful.

In addition, the primary care practitioner should be able to relate this topic to other aspects of the patient's wellbeing which may be relevant – whether this is their need for a change in contraception, their recent binge-drinking or a history of domestic violence.

Each of these steps will be discussed in turn. With this overview, the GP or practice nurse is then in a position to decide when referral to GUM is indicated, and, if it is, they will be able to explain to the patient why.

Which infections are sexually transmissible, and which are not?

It is important for GPs and practice nurses to be clear in their minds about which infections are usually or invariably sexually transmitted and which are not. This knowledge should underpin discussions with patients about which tests to take, how to interpret results and how to manage their condition.

GPs and practice nurses need to be confident about which infections are:

- not sexually transmissible
- sexually transmissible *and* transmissible by other routes
- solely sexually transmitted.

It is essential to be clear about this, in order that:

- patients are clear about how they may have acquired the infection, and how they can protect themselves and others in the future
- referral options are appropriate.

Genital infections *not* managed as sexually transmissible

There are a number of genital infections and conditions which cause confusion. It is essential that patients who are *not* at risk of STIs are not inadvertently told they have one, when they haven't. Those infections that are *not* managed as sexually transmitted include:

- Bacterial vaginosis.
- Candida (this arises spontaneously – treatment of the partner rarely prevents recurrence).
- Gardnerella vaginalis.
- Haemolytic streptococcus Group B.

Organisms which are commonly sexually transmitted

Certain infections are commonly sexually transmitted (see list below). Risks of the sexual transmission of different organisms may vary. For example, pubic lice can be transmitted by close genital contact despite careful use of a condom. However, risk of transmission of gonorrhoea is greatly reduced (if not eliminated) where condom use is 'ideal'.

If these organisms are found because of another route of transmission (for example, vertical transmission of gonorrhoea leading to conjunctivitis in a baby) then clinical management still needs to take into account sexual transmission (for example, management of the mother and her sexual contact(s)).

Infections which are often sexually transmitted include:

- Chlamydia trachomatis.
- Neisseria gonorrhoea.
- Herpes simplex viruses (HSV I and II).
- HIV.
- Hepatitis B.
- Human papilloma virus (HPV).
- Pubic lice.
- Treponema pallidum (syphilis).

- Trichomonas vaginalis (TV).

- Mycoplasma genitalum.

In addition, there is significant sexual transmission of:

- Hepatitis A.

- Scabies.

Hepatitis C is rarely sexually transmitted.

Recognising that an STI may be present

Symptomatic patients

There is a wealth of both direct and indirect evidence that we are seeing people with symptoms of STIs in primary care. One study based at a 'walk-in' GUM clinic in London found that 40 per cent of attenders found to have an STI had already been seen in primary care for their problem[9]. Those who had attended primary care had a longer symptom-to-treatment interval than patients who presented directly to the GUM clinic. If patients are unaware that their symptoms could be caused by an STI, they will present in primary care, not GUM. Hence, improvement in GU access will not improve symptom-to-treatment intervals for this group.

GPs therefore need to have an excellent understanding of the diverse ways that STIs can present. An old-fashioned model relying more or less on the symptoms of urethral or vaginal discharge will not suffice. Consider which STIs may lead patients to present with the following problems – the numbers in brackets indicate the *minimum* number of sexually transmitted infective agents you should be able to think of.

persistent conjunctivitis in a young adult (1)
arthralgia (2)
glandular fever-like illness (1)
dysuria in men (3)
intermenstrual bleeding (1)
cystitis-like symptoms in women (2)
genital ulcers (2)
sterile pyuria (white cells but no organism cultured) (1)
epididymitis or orchitis (1)
vaginal discharge (3 STIs)
hard-to-treat seborrhoeic dermatitis (1)

right upper quadrant (RUQ) pain in women (1)

jaundice (2)

bruise-like lesions on skin (1)

menorrhagia (1)

molluscum contagiosum in adults (1)

atypical chest infections (1)

post-coital bleeding (1)

pelvic inflammatory disease (2)

Check the symptom grid on page 174 for answers. Any that are missing may be found in Chapter 7.

This diversity of symptoms leads to a need for differential diagnosis in the patients concerned. There are often other possible causes for their symptoms that are not related to STIs. Indeed some of our patients with symptoms such as these may be at no risk at all of having an STI. The process of differential diagnosis is aided by taking a history to assess risk for STI. This is discussed in Chapter 2.

Babies with symptoms because of vertical transmission of infection

STIs may also be vertically transmitted from mother to baby in pregnancy or in the birth canal, and GPs will sometimes see the consequences of this. Trichomonas vaginalis may be associated with preterm birth. Antenatal detection of some infections is the priority, coupled with appropriate interventions to reduce or eliminate risk of transmission to the baby. This is the case, for example, for hepatitis B, HIV and genital herpes. The GP may therefore be cushioned from the need to detect these infections in babies – at least where antenatal testing is comprehensive for HIV and hepatitis B. However, other infections are likely to present in primary care:

- chlamydia characteristically causes a mild persistent conjunctivitis or 'sticky eye', which may be indistinguishable clinically from a blocked tear duct
- gonorrhoea generally causes a more severe conjunctivitis in neonates
- chlamydia can cause a pneumonia in neonates
- HPV can cause laryngeal papillomatosis in babies.

Incidental findings from urine samples or smears

It is possible in primary care to come across STIs as an incidental finding:

- A mid-stream urine specimen (MSU) showing white cells with no organisms grown (especially in a young, fit, person, whether male or female) is most likely to be caused by chlamydia. This possibility should be explored with the patient with a view to testing. Some labs automatically test specimens showing sterile pyuria for chlamydia, but (depending upon the test they use) this may not be as effective in detecting chlamydia infection as a genital swab (see page 166). In men with sterile pyuria not found to have chlamydia a diagnosis of non-specific urethritis (NSU) is highly likely.

- HPV causes a characteristic appearance (poikilocytosis) on smears that some (but not all) cytology labs will report. If it is reported, this finding should be discussed with the patient, although bear in mind that HPV is extremely common and may well have been present for several years. It may or may not be appropriate to offer her a test for chlamydia, or offer advice as to how she might protect her sexual health in the future.

- Trichomonas vaginalis reported on smears *may not be reliable*; some labs only mean 'TV-like' organisms, rather than TV itself. Talk to the patient and see if they have any symptoms. Do an STI risk assessment and offer an appropriate test for TV as required.

Asymptomatic patients

All sexually transmissible infections can be transmitted from someone who has *no* symptoms. This is as true of herpes and gonorrhoea as it is of chlamydia and HIV.

Asymptomatic patients with STIs will be attending primary care. The National Chlamydia Screening Pilots in Portsmouth and Wirrall[10] offered chlamydia tests to all attenders aged 16 to 24 in GUM, young people's services and primary care. Those attending primary care made up the biggest proportion of total positive results, simply because of the scale of the clinical service. Prevalence rates in primary care in this study were shown to be just under 9 per cent – only slightly lower than in the other services. People with undiagnosed HIV infection will of course be attending primary care[11], and some of them will have no symptoms that are caused by their HIV infection.

Knowing the important clinical consequences of individual STIs

GPs and practice nurses should be familiar with the clinical consequences of individual STIs, many of which can have serious health implications. Health professionals should be able to give clear information to any patients who are considering a test for (or have been found to have) an infection. It is important that the consequences of *untreated* infection are distinguished from the consequences of *treated* infections (for example, treatment for HIV is highly effective, but does not eliminate the organism). It is often possible to be reassuring with patients and point out that it is much better to know about the infection than not to know about it. This is particularly true of HIV and chlamydia.

Confirming the diagnosis

The diagnosis of an STI depends upon:

- clinical diagnosis
- microbiological diagnosis.

Some infections are diagnosed solely on a clinical basis (for example, genital warts, pubic lice or a new presentation of AIDS requiring admission). In other situations there may be strong, or subtle, clinical clues, but microbiological confirmation is very helpful (genital herpes, gonorrhoea or HIV disease). Many infections may be asymptomatic and diagnosed *solely* by tests (for example, opportunistic HIV or chlamydia testing).

Clinical diagnosis

GPs with the clinical skills to recognise diagnostic presentations of STIs (for example, typical genital warts, genital herpes or pubic lice) may sometimes be able to avoid referring the patient on. Clinical teaching with a primary care focus and some experience in GUM will help GPs to consolidate their clinical skills. Some texts have photographs which are of value (see Further information, page 179).

Table 6.2 (page 174) helps clinicians to identify which symptoms and clinical findings may be caused by STIs, and which may give diagnostic catches.

Microbiological diagnosis

The 'near patient' microbiology lab in many GUM clinics continues to have a role, but this has lessened as diagnostic techniques have improved and become less reliant on microscopy. In primary care, these improvements in diagnostic techniques have great potential, although some microbiology labs are quicker to make progress than others.

Clinicians in primary care need to know, as far as possible:

- which tests are available to them (and which *should* be available to them)
- how soon after infection a given test is likely to become positive
- what specimens are best collected for which clinical situation
- how best to store and to transport samples
- how to interpret test results.

Some points are made below on each of these issues, although it is difficult to give an overview when local variations are so marked. Perhaps the single most important step is to initiate a dialogue with your local microbiologist about each of the above issues. Your lab should be able to provide you with some information about the sensitivity and specificity of the tests provided, to help you interpret your results.

Which tests are available for which infections? How should they be interpreted?

The clinician caring for, for example, a symptomatic patient who is at risk of chlamydia requires a test which has, above all, a high sensitivity and specificity. Tests selected for population screening programmes may prioritise different characteristics. For instance, the ability for the patient to collect the specimen themselves may increase uptake of a screening programme significantly, and so override the effect of a decrease in sensitivity. Primary care clinicians should have available the tests that best suit their needs.

How soon after a patient has been infected is a given test likely to become positive?

The minimum time lapse between becoming infected and the likely detection of infection by most *swab-based* tests (as distinct from blood tests) is unclear. Newer DNA-based techniques are likely to be more sensitive in very early infection. Antibodies take time to develop after the infection has been acquired, and the time taken from infection until the test becomes positive is known as the window period. Where available, guidance is given below underneath the individual tests discussed. Advice should be sought if you are in doubt. If uncertainty remains, tests should be repeated.

Nucleic acid amplification tests (NAATs)

These highly sensitive and specific tests present hope of transforming the detection of STIs, and indeed have already done so for chlamydia (although many laboratories still fail to provide such tests). DNA-based tests for gonorrhoea are now also emerging. The tests are based on amplification of genetic material specific to a given organism. Examples include polymerase chain reaction (PCR) and strand displacement amplification (SDA).

DNA-based tests are capable of detecting genetic material from dead organisms, which may mean that specimens collected in a practice on a Friday evening could still yield positive results. However, dead material may of course also lead to a false positive result from a patient who has recently been successfully treated – unless four weeks have been allowed to lapse for the dead organisms to clear.

Increasingly these tests enable organisms to be detected from samples collected in less invasive ways, most notably chlamydia on vulval wipes or urine tests which may be self-collected.

Microscopy

Microscopy is not available or realistic for many practices. In GUM it enables immediate diagnosis of gonorrhoea, Trichomonas vaginalis, non-specific urethritis (NSU) and, along with the other diagnostic features, bacterial vaginosis (BV). Gonorrhoea culture will still be required to check sensitivities.

Non-specific urethritis (NSU) is diagnosed by microscopy in GUM. The diagnosis of NSU in primary care is more difficult. If a male patient has dysuria it may be most appropriate to exclude other possible STIs by taking tests for other STIs such as gonorrhoea and chlamydia. A urine specimen should also be sent to look for sterile pyuria (and rule out a urinary tract infection – more likely in older patients). If no organisms are detected on the swab (and if sterile pyuria is detected on a urine specimen) then manage as NSU or refer to GUM for partner notification. Follow up is needed to ensure that sterile pyuria has resolved in order to exclude rare causes such as renal TB.

Culture

Bacterial and other culture:

- Gonorrhoea. This is considered a fragile organism to transport and culture, but it is possible to detect regularly in primary care in higher prevalence areas. Check with your lab which culture medium is preferred, as this varies.

- Trichomonas vaginalis.

- Candida, haemolytic streptococcus group B and Gardnerella vaginalis – among other organisms – can also be detected by culture.

Chlamydia culture: This is insufficiently sensitive and has been superceded by DNA amplification techniques.

Genital herpes culture: Viruses are intracellular, and cells from the base of an ulcer need to be obtained on the swab. The sampling techniques for viral culture differ from other swabs in two ways. First, the swab should be dipped in the medium *before* being rubbed over the ulcer. Second, the chances of successful culture are improved if *two* swab tips (as opposed to just one) are placed in the same culture medium – that is, carry out the swab procedure *twice* using only one bottle of medium.

Enzyme-linked immunosorbent assay (ELISA)

This used to be the mainstay of chlamydia diagnosis. Earlier versions of this test were cheap but not very sensitive or specific. Newer generations are significantly better. Clinicians should discuss the sensitivity and specificity of any test provided. They should also check whether additional confirmatory tests are required if results are positive in order to exclude false positives.

Antibody tests on blood

Antibody tests are used to detect some infections. The time taken for them to become positive, following infection, is known as the window period.

- HIV (for more details on the interpretation of HIV tests, see Chapter 7).

- Hepatitis A (window period seven weeks).

- Hepatitis B (window period six weeks to six months). For more details on the interpretation of hepatitis results, see Further information, page 179, and the sample hepatitis B guidance, page 182).

- Hepatitis C (window period usually three months, but may be up to nine months).

Tests for syphilis

Syphilis belongs to a group of diseases caused by organisms of the Treponema family.

Blood tests for syphilis can be divided into two groups:

- **Non-treponemal tests**, which detect non-specific treponemal antibody. These include VDRL and RPR tests.

- **Treponemal tests**, which detect specific treponemal antibody. These include TPHA, FTA-abs and EIA tests.

Tests used vary between laboratories; tests may not become positive for up to three months.

If treponemal antibody is detected by a screening test, then a second confirmatory test, on the same sample, will be undertaken. This second test would have a greater specificity than, and use a different method from, the initial test, to avoid false positive results.

If this sample tests positive after both tests, then a second sample should be taken to confirm the results from the first specimen.

What specimens are best collected from which clinical sites?

This depends on the organism being considered and also the clinical picture.

Chlamydia commonly infects endocervical and urethral cells, and the samples collected reflect this. However, highly sensitive tests may be conducted on, for example, vulval wipes. Chlamydia may infect the conjunctiva or more rarely the pharynx and elsewhere (for example, it is occasionally isolated from inflamed joints).

Gonorrhoea is present in discharge from the infected area, and so the clinical picture should guide sampling for culture. The discharge is usually emerging from the cervical os in women and from the urethra in men. Gonorrhoea may also cause neonatal conjunctivitis and discharge from the eye which will need to be sampled. It may occasionally cause rectal discharge, pharyngeal infection or infection elsewhere. Gonorrhoea is not thought to survive in the vagina, although future generations of diagnostic test may enable testing to be conducted on high vaginal swabs, vulval wipes or urine samples.

Trichomonas vaginalis causes a vaginal infection in women, and urethral in men.

In women with possible genital infection, take three specimens:

- a high vaginal swab to collect discharge (TV and other vaginal infections)
- an endocervical swab to collect discharge (gonorrhoea).This is generally taken *before* any endocervical swab for chlamydia
- the available test for genital chlamydia – commonly a swab to collect endocervical cells (discharge should be removed first).

In primary care, urethral and rectal swabs are rarely required from women. However, you may need to consider this if no infection is detected on genital swabs but symptoms relate to the urethra or rectum.

In men with possible genital infection, take the following specimens:

- a urethral swab to collect discharge (TV, gonorrhoea) is taken first
- the available test for genital chlamydia – often a swab to collect urethral cells
- a urine specimen may be taken to look for sterile pyuria as evidence of NSU or to exclude urinary tract infection.

In persistent conjunctivitis where an STI may be a cause, take:

- a swab to collect discharge from the eye for gonorrhoea

- a sample to collect conjunctival cells for chlamydia – although labs may tell you that their tests are not well-validated for this type of sample. If there is a problem, it is more likely to be with false negatives that with false positives.

Other sites may occasionally need to be sampled if the clinical picture dictates. These include the throat, or rectum (referral to GUM may be helpful in the latter instance). However, newer tests may not be validated for these sites, and so it may be necessary to discuss which test to use with your microbiologist.

Storing and transporting samples

In the absence of good evidence as to the best ways to store specimens from primary care, practices should ensure that all samples are refrigerated shortly after being taken. Generally, samples for culture should be transported to the lab as soon as possible (DNA-based techniques are more tolerant). Nevertheless, organisms can sometimes be cultured even when there has been significant delay. This includes gonorrhoea, which is considered fragile.

Screening for other infections, once an STI diagnosis is confirmed

Because STIs are commonly found in conjunction with other STIs, the confirmation of one infection should be followed by further tests for other infections. Whether the diagnosis is pubic lice, Trichomonas vaginalis or genital warts, the following tests (if they have not already been done) should be offered to the patient:

- chlamydia
- gonorrhoea
- HIV
- hepatitis B
- syphilis.

If a patient does not attend GUM, the GP or practice nurse should consider offering these tests to a patient found to have an STI.

It is important to note the following clinical points:

- If culture was positive for an organism (for example Trichomonas vaginalis), then this organism may have overgrown other culture specimens taken at the same time (for example gonorrhoea); these tests may therefore need to be repeated after treatment.
- A clinical diagnosis of an uncomfortable condition such as herpes may require the deferral of other investigations, until the pain has settled.

Full and appropriate treatment

Many infections respond to antibiotic or antiviral drugs. Currently recommended treatment for individual infections is readily available from a number of sources (see Further information, page 179). If a patient has a minor STI but will not attend GUM (or says they will and then does not attend), then it may be appropriate for GPs to arrange management. If a patient with gonorrhoea fails or refuses to attend GUM then it may be a priority to arrange treatment according to recent guidelines rather than let the infection remain untreated. Other aspects of management discussed here (such as testing for other infections and partner notification) will also need to be considered.

Advice and information for the patient

The patient with an STI needs to understand the following points:

Transmission and prevention of transmission

- How the infection can be transmitted.
- That many infections can be present for a significant length of time before being detected (years in the case of chlamydia and HIV).
- How long to abstain from sexual intercourse after treatment.
- How to protect him/herself from infection in the future.
- The importance of treating sexual contacts.
- That the patient's sexual contact/s may be unaware that they [the contact] have or had an infection.
- Where the patient's sexual contact/s can get treatment.

The medication

- The effects of an untreated infection.
- How to take the medication.
- The importance of completing the course.
- Possible side effects.
- What the patient should do if they have not managed to complete the course of treatment for any reason.

Test of cure (see When are tests of cure indicated, page 171)

- Whether it is indicated.
- When it should be done.

If the patient is referred for further care

- When and where to attend.

- What to expect from that service.

This may also be the appropriate time to consider or revisit other aspects of sexual health, such as risk of unwanted pregnancy in heterosexual patients, or whether women are up-to-date with cervical screening.

Written information

Try to back up the information given to the patient with written resources where possible. **fpa** has produced a series of leaflets for the public on STIs. For details, see Further information, page 179.

Partner notification

There is often misunderstanding about partner notification. There is evidence that practice nurses working in practices participating in a chlamydia screening study, who have undergone brief additional training, are as good at supporting successful partner notification as health advisers[12]. Some people hold unrealistic views of the lengths that will be gone to in order to trace a contact. In addition, assumptions are made that it is required for all STIs. In fact, active attempts are only made to trace sexual contacts of patients with infections for which there are:

- significant implications for health

- effective treatment or prevention strategies.

Partner notification is *not* carried out for the following infections:

- genital warts or HPV infection

- genital herpes.

This is because treatments affect symptoms only. Other outcomes are not significantly affected.

Treatment of *current partner only* can be offered for:

- Trichomonas vaginalis

- pubic lice

- scabies.

This is done in order to prevent reinfection of the index patient. These infections do not have significant consequences to health, and formal partner notification is not carried out.

Partner notification *is* conducted for infections which have serious consequences but which are eradicated or improved by treatment or clinical monitoring. Partner notification is attempted for the following infections:

- gonorrhoea
- chlamydia
- NSU (although no organism has been identified)
- PID
- HIV
- syphilis
- hepatitis B.

The criteria for how far back contacts are traced vary from infection to infection (see Table 6.1 below). If relevant information on contacts is not available *("I think he was called John and I met him in a nightclub. No, I don't know any more about him")*, then no further attempt will be made to track the contact. This is the case even when the infection is HIV.

Partner notification is conducted by health advisers, generally based in GUM clinics, although new models are being explored. There are a number of ways of conducting partner notification, including asking the patient him/herself to inform partners, or contacting partners by phone or letter. For details on the evidence of the effectiveness of different methods of partner notification, see Clinical Evidence[13].

Table 6.1:

Which contacts require notification and treatment?

Infection	Treat sexual contacts within preceding:
Gonorrhoea	
Men with symptoms	2 weeks
Asymptomatic men	3 months
All women	3 months
Chlamydia	
Men with symptoms	1 month
Asymptomatic men	6 months
All women	6 months

NSU	
Symptomatic	1 month
Asymptomatic	6 months
PID	Test all male partners within 6 months for chlamydia and gonorrhoea
HIV Syphilis Hepatitis B Hepatitis C	Patients are advised that current and past sexual partners should be informed. The period of 'look back' can vary enormously, depending on whether it is a recent infection, or may have been acquired many years previously.

When are tests of cure indicated?

Tests of cure (TOC), or repeat tests, are indicated:

- When the patient has had chlamydia treated with erythromycin (usually because she is or may be pregnant). Erythromycin is a less effective treatment for chlamydia and TOC is required even if the patient has complied fully with their management.

- If there is suspected treatment failure, treatment non-compliance or reinfection (gonorrhoea has significant problems with antibiotic resistance; TV sometimes requires a second course of antibiotics).

- When a culture has grown an organism (for example, TV) that may have overgrown, and so masked, more fragile organisms (for example, gonorrhoea). This situation should be considered if symptoms have not resolved following treatment.

REFERRAL TO GUM

There is good evidence that many patients with STIs present first in primary care[14,15]. However, referral on to GUM from primary care often remains informal, for example a verbal recommendation to the patient to attend GUM, perhaps accompanied by a leaflet. This is distinct from referrals on for a specialist opinion in other clinical specialties, when a referral letter will be sent via post, email or fax.

Why has this informal referral process arisen?

It is unclear. GUM is an open access service: patients can self-refer. It may be that GPs are simply using this attribute in order to avoid writing a referral letter. Alternatively GPs may feel that a written record of a GUM referral may somehow jeopardise confidentiality for the patient (although presumably a record of the original consultation is kept). These fears about confidentiality may reflect a concern that, because GUM is an open access confidential service, patients have a 'right' to conceal STI care from their GP. In addition, GPs may be concerned that mention of an STI on medical reports for insurance purposes could jeopardise the patient's chances of obtaining insurance.

Are these confidentiality concerns founded?

GPs and GUM clinics may be being inappropriately coy about confidentiality issues. One study showed that 61 out of 75 GUM patients were happy for the GUM clinic to write to their GP *whether originally referred by the GP or not* – and they delivered the letter themselves[16]. Another study found that anxieties about confidentiality in primary care did not appear to be a worry for more than a small minority of patients[17]. GPs concerned about insurance reports may draw some reassurance from a recent BMA and insurance industry collaboration to improve the consistency and relevance of information collected for insurance purposes (www.bma.org. uk). This indicates that episodes of most STIs can be ignored for the purposes of insurance medical reports. GPs should only complete insurance reports which adhere to the agreed BMA format and also the agreed standard of patient consent.

Non-attendance at GUM and the role of the GP

It is a fact that a proportion of patients referred on to *any* speciality will not attend their appointment. For patients in some areas, referral to GUM may represent a round trip covering many miles and this may be daunting or impossible for a young person. The issue of non-attendance following referral to GUM is under-researched, although there is limited evidence that rates may be particularly high[18,19]. In addition, a small proportion of patients say to their primary care clinician that they will not attend a GUM clinic.

The GP who has a good overview of how STIs are managed, is in a much better position to help patients to understand when and why GUM attendance is essential for their care. This may increase patients' motivation to attend – especially if their symptoms have settled and are no longer a motivating factor (whether or not the infection has been eradicated).

The costs to quality of care of using informal referral

There are a number of problems which arise when informal referral to a service is used.

A failure of the system to detect non-attendance and hence respond to it

A lack of a proper referral system means that GUM staff will be unaware that a patient failed to attend, and so cannot notify the GP. No one will 'chase up' the patient, who may continue to spread an untreated infection, or simply become re-infected because their partner was not treated.

A failure of clinical dialogue between two doctors may lead to poor care

A referral letter and reply ensure that important points of the patient's clinical care can be highlighted in the normal way, for example, notification of drug allergies or prescribed medication.

A missed opportunity to inform and educate GPs about important clinical conditions

Letters from specialists are important sources of information and education for GPs on the whole spectrum of conditions. GUM should be no exception.

A missed opportunity to monitor and improve service design

There is currently a crisis in provision of GUM services, with some services so overstretched that they are turning patients away[20]. Improved levels of knowledge and care in primary care could help to avoid unnecessary referrals and play a part in alleviating the pressure on the specialist services. If it is not known how many GUM patients are referred from primary care, how can the impact of relevant change and development in either of these services be monitored?

Proposals for the future

It is time for the referral interface with GUM to be normalised. There is a need to adopt the same standards for referral to GUM from primary care as for other specialities. This would lead to a model something like this:

- The GP understands who should be referred to GUM, what can be offered there for the common infections, and what is urgent.
- A normal quality referral letter is written by the GP, one copy of which goes directly to the GUM clinic by an agreed route (post, fax or electronically). The letter should include contact details as agreed with the patient.
- The GUM clinic gives the patient either an urgent or routine appointment.
- If the patient fails to attend, there should be an agreed procedure, for example the GP is notified by the clinic; or the clinic contacts the patient directly by mobile.

- The GUM clinic writes to the GP after each clinic attendance.

For practices able to provide a high quality of STI diagnosis and care, it may be valuable to explore outreach models of partner notification so that referrals to GUM can prioritise those most in need of an expert clinical opinion.

Table 6.2:

Some symptoms which may suggest more common STIs (excluding HIV, and many presentations of syphilis, see Further information, page 179)

Symptoms and signs	Syndromes or underlying condition if symptom is caused by an STI	Possible causes
Women only		
Vaginal bleeding irregularities *Post coital bleeding* *Intermenstrual bleeding* *Menorrhagia*	Cervicitis Endometritis	Chlamydia *Several non-STI causes may need to be excluded*
Abdominal pain Pelvic pain Deep dyspareunia Fever Vaginal discharge *Symptoms and signs may be mild* *Not all of these symptoms may be present in PID*	Pelvic inflammatory disease Salpingitis Curtis Fitz-Hugh syndrome *(peri-hepatitis – chlamydia only)* Peri-appendicitis *(chlamydia only)*	Chlamydia Gonorrhoea *Non-STI causes include appendicitis, cholecystitis.*
Vaginal discharge		Gonorrhoea Trichomonas vaginalis Chlamydia *(rarely – some think chlamydia does not cause discharge)* *Non-STI causes include BV, candida and many other conditions*
Men only		
Urethral discharge		Gonorrhoea Chlamydia Trichomonas vaginalis *Non STI causes*
Pain in testicle or over epididymis	Epididymo-orchitis	Chlamydia *Non-STI causes including infections*

Symptoms and signs	Syndromes or underlying condition if symptom is caused by an STI	Possible causes
Women and men		
Dysuria Urinary frequency	i) Urethritis	Chlamydia NSU (men) Gonorrhoea Genital herpes *Non STI causes include urinary tract infection, candida, urethral stricture or trauma*
	ii) Sexually acquired reactive arthritis (SARA) See below	ii) SARA – see below
Genital ulceration i) painful ii) usually painless and solitary		i) Genital herpes, possibly TV ii) Syphilis Could patient have STI endemic to third world such as chancroid? *Non-STI causes include candida, Behcets, drug eruptions and several general dermatological conditions*
Genital lumps	i) Warts	i) Genital warts (HPV) *Non-STI causes may be multiple, but genital warts usually have a characteristic appearance*
	ii) Rarely Condylomata lata	ii) Syphilis can cause an appearance similar to multiple genital warts
Genital itching		Pubic lice Occasionally genital herpes *Non-STI causes include candida and dermatological conditions*
Inguinal Lymphadenopathy	Pelvic Inflammatory Disease	Chlamydia (including Lymphogranuloma venereum serovars) Gonorrhoea Herpes *Multiple non STI causes*
Proctitis		Gonorrhoea Lymphogranuloma venereum

Symptoms and signs	Syndromes or underlying condition if symptom is caused by an STI	Possible causes
Sterile pyuria (white cells on MSU but no organism identified)		Chlamydia NSU (men) *Non-STI causes are rare and include renal stones or renal TB*
Sexually acquired reactive arthritis (SARA): Urethritis Conjunctivitis Joint pain (one or few, lower limb) More rarely iritis; rash on palms and soles (pustular psoriasis); mouth ulcers; erythema nodosum	SARA *Reactive arthritis due to enteric infections as opposed to STIs may cause identical symptoms – including urethritis*	Chlamydia Gonorrhoea *Non-STI causes for reactive arthritis include enteric infections such as campylobacter or salmonella.*
Rash on soles of feet (or rarely palms)	i) Pustular psoriasis on the soles (Keratoderma Blennorrhagica *associated with SARA, see above*) ii) Syphilis	i) see above ii) Syphilis
Jaundice		Hepatitis A, B or C *Multiple non-STI causes*
Joint pains	i) Local infection ii) SARA *(see above)*	Chlamydia Gonorrhoea *Multiple non-STI causes* ii) See above
Discharge from eye Discomfort in eye	i) Conjunctivitis ii) SARA *(see above)*	i) Chlamydia Gonorrhoea (neonates only) *Multiple non-STI causes* ii) See above

NB Syphilis and HIV are both 'great imitators' and present in an enormous variety of ways that cannot be covered here – see Further information, page 179, for details of how HIV presents.

SUPPORTING QUALITY AND AUDIT IN PRIMARY CARE

Current clinical guidelines for STI management are not written for the primary care setting. Many of the guidelines which are available through the websites given in Further information (page 179) are also cumbersome to use. The introduction of 'enhanced services' in sexual health through the current GMS Contract for GPs[21] may start to focus primary care trusts and boards on data collection and quality

THE HANDBOOK OF SEXUAL HEALTH IN PRIMARY CARE

measures for STI diagnosis and management in primary care. This may lead to the development of resources that are centred on the primary care context.

Practices wishing to provide high quality sexual health care should start with the development of a protocol that suits their needs, and then provide the training required to implement it. The sources below are a starting point, but practices will have to consider aspects particular to their context. For example, who should the practices prioritise when offering STI or HIV tests? Some aspects of this are addressed in Chapter 2 on sexual history-taking. Similarly, the issue of referral to GUM should be addressed and will need to be discussed with your local GUM service. An example of hepatitis B testing and immunisation protocol for primary care is included in Annex 1.

With a protocol in place it then becomes possible for the primary care team to agree what data they wish to collect and audit, and to select the Read codes which are to be used. Computer templates can also be used to support this process.

Key messages

- Many prevalent STIs can be present with no symptoms.
- The symptoms of STIs are diverse and may be subtle or insidious – be sure not to limit recognition only to those patients with discharge.
- High quality STI testing is possible in the primary care context, although clinicians may need to review their current practice and start a constructive dialogue with their pathology laboratory.

References

1. Health Protection Agency. *Renewing the Focus: HIV and Other Sexually Transmitted Infections in the United Kingdom in 2002*. Annual Report, November 2003. http://www.hpa.org.uk

2. House of Commons Health Committee. *Sexual Health.* Third report of session 2002–2003. HC69–1, London: The Stationery Office 2003.

3. See note 2 above.

4. Department of Health, *National Strategy for Sexual Health and HIV.* London: Department of Health 2001

5. Pimenta J, Catchpole M and Rogers P et al. Opportunistic screening for genital chlamydial infection. II: Prevalence among health care attenders, outcome, and evaluation of positive cases. *Sexually Transmitted Infections*, vol 79, no 1, 2003, pp22–27.

6. Cassell J et al. Treating sexually transmitted infections in primary care: a missed opportunity? *Sexually Transmitted Infections*, vol 79, no 2, 2003, pp134–36.

7. See note 2 above.

8. British Medical Association (BMA) and NHS Confederation, *Investing in General Practice: The New General Medical Services Contract.* London: NHS Confederation and BMA 2003.

9. See note 6 above.

10. See note 5 above.

11. Madge S et al. Access to medical care one year prior to diagnosis in 100 HIV-positive women. *Family Practice*, vol 14, no 3, 1997, pp255–257.

12. Low N et al. Partner Notification of Chlamydia Infection in Primary Care: Randomised Controlled Trial and Analysis of Resource Use. *BMJ*, vol 322, no 7532, 2006, pp14–18. Markham W et al. Sexual health care training needs of GP trainers: a regional survey. *Journal of Family Planning and Reproductive Health Care*, vol 31, no 3, 2005, pp213–18.

13. *Clinical Evidence*. BMJ Publishing. http://www.clinicalevidence.com

14. See note 6 above.

15. Clutterbuck D and Ross D. Sources of information on genitourinary medicine clinics. *International Journal of STD and AIDS*, vol 8, no 8, 1997, p532.

16. Winceslaus J, Blount J and Cryer C. Sexually transmitted diseases and communications with general practitioners. *Sexually Transmitted Infections*, vol 75, no 1, 1999, pp45–48.

17. See note 6 above.

18. Tobin J et al. Clinical audit of the process of referral to genitourinary medicine of patients found to be chlamydia positive in a family planning service. *British Journal of Family Planning*, vol 24, no 4, 1999, pp160–63.

19. Matthews P, Fletcher J and Allen E. *An investigation into the management of sexually transmitted diseases in primary care.* Report to NHSE West Midlands (locally organised research scheme) 2000.

20. See note 2 above.

21. See note 8 above.

Further information

General texts on STIs

Donovan B. Sexually transmissible infections other than HIV. *The Lancet*, vol 363, pp545–56.

Adler M. *ABC of Sexually Transmitted Infections* (5th edition). BMJ Books, 2004.

Adler M. *ABC of AIDS* (5th edition). BMJ Books, 2001.

Kumar P and Clarke M. *Clinical Medicine*. Balliere Tindall, 2002.

fpa leaflets on STIs

- *Your sexual health – where to go for help and advice*
- *Chlamydia*
- *Genital herpes*
- *Genital warts*
- *Gonorrhoea*
- *HIV*
- *Pubic lice and scabies*
- *Syphilis*
- *Trichomonas vaginalis*
- *Vaginal infections (thrush and BV)*

Available from **fpa**
Tel: 0845 122 8600
Fax: 0845 123 2349
Email: fpadirect@fpa.org.uk
www.fpa.org.uk

Two articles debating the role and priorities of GUM clinics in the UK

Bradbeer C and Meers A. STI services in the United Kingdom: how shall we cope? *Sexually Transmitted Infections,* vol 79, 2003, pp435–38.

Carne C. STI services in the United Kingdom: a way forward. *Sexually Transmitted Infections,* vol 79, 2003, pp439–41.

Useful websites

Notes on use of the websites

A resource tailored to your own needs (but based on national guidelines) may be much more suitable for quick reference than many of the full guidelines given below (see Supporting quality and audit in primary care, page 176).

The British Association of Sexual Health and HIV (BASHH) was formerly the Medical Society for the study of Venereal Diseases (MSSVD).

Individual infections and conditions	Background information	Epidemiology	Treatment
Bacterial vaginosis	www.prodigy.nhs.uk	www.hpa.org.uk	www.bashh.org
Candida	www.prodigy.nhs.uk	www.hpa.org.uk	www.bashh.org
Chlamydia (also for Lymphogranuloma venereum)	www.chlamydiae.com www.prodigy.nhs.uk	www.hpa.org.uk	www.bashh.org
Gardnerella vaginalis	Normal commensal, but see bacterial vaginosis		
Genital herpes	www.herpesalliance.org www.prodigy.nhs.uk	www.hpa.org.uk	www.bashh.org
Genital warts	www.prodigy.nhs.uk www.niaid.nih.gov (USA)	www.hpa.org.uk	www.bashh.org
Gonorrhoea	www.sexualhealthmatters.com (vol 3 issue 3) www.nelh.nhs.uk (search medical dictionaries) www.hpa.org.uk	www.hpa.org.uk	www.bashh.org
Haemolytic streptococcus Group B	www.gbss.org.uk www.hpa.org.uk www.cdc.gov (USA)		www.rcog.org.uk www.bashh.org www.cdc.gov
Hepatitis A	www.britishlivertrust.org.uk	www.hpa.org.uk	www.bashh.org
Hepatitis B	www.britishlivertrust.org.uk	www.hpa.org.uk	www.bashh.org
Hepatitis C	www.hepc.org.uk www.britishlivertrust.org.uk	www.hpa.org.uk	www.nice.org.uk
Human papilloma virus – see genital warts		www.hpa.org.uk	

Individual infections and conditions	Background information	Epidemiology	Treatment
HIV	www.aidsmap.com	www.hpa.org.uk	www.bhiva.org www.aidsmap.com
Non-specific urethritis	www.prodigy.nhs.uk	www.hpa.org.uk	www.bashh.org
Pelvic inflammatory disease	www.prodigy.nhs.uk		www.bashh.org
Pubic lice	www.prodigy.nhs.uk	www.hpa.org.uk	www.bashh.org
Sexually acquired reactive arthritis (Reiter's Syndrome)	www.emedicine.com/emerg/topic498.htm		www.bashh.org
Scabies	www.prodigy.nhs.uk	www.hpa.org.uk	www.bashh.org
Syphilis	www.hpa.org.uk www.niaid.nih.gov (USA)	www.hpa.org.uk	www.bashh.org
Trichomonas vaginalis	www.prodigy.nhs.uk	www.hpa.org.uk	www.bashh.org

Annex 1

HEPATITIS B TESTING AND IMMUNISATION GUIDANCE

Red Chimneys Practice

Leads[1]
Dr May Black
Ms Hazel Grey

External reviewer[2]
Dr X Pert

Aims

- To identify people at risk of hepatitis B with a view to offering them testing.
- To increase awareness of hepatitis B and how it is transmitted.
- To increase detection of hepatitis B in those at risk.
- To provide a non-judgemental service.

Who to test for hepatitis B immunity (hepatitis B surface antibody)

These people are at highest risk of *prior* hepatitis B infection:

- born in an endemic country (Far East, Africa, Indian sub-continent, Caribbean)
- IVDU – shared works (not just needles)
- been in prison/institution
- multiple sexual partners (including sex workers)
- risky sexual contact (higher if man who has sex with men)
- HIV positive
- victim of sexual assault
- partner born in endemic country, IVDU or potentially any of the above.

These groups may be at higher risk and thus benefit from immunisation:

- occupational risk

1. Appropriate clinical members of the team
2. Usually a local specialist

- health care workers
- prison/institution workers
- emergency service employees
- international travellers
- family and sexual contacts of infected patients.

Don't deter anyone who requests a test

Issues to discuss
- Recent risks – (up to six months) – if significant, get advice re: appropriate testing and role of post-exposure procedure.
- Risk minimisation.
- Implications for partners/family/work if current infection identified.
- (Sometimes) other blood borne viruses, for example, HIV.

Contraindications to immunisation
- Severe febrile illness – rearrange for when well.
- Known sensitivity to vaccine.
- Manufacturers list pregnancy as a contraindication: seek advice.

Blood sampling
- Take blood sample in appropriate tube.
- Enter *either* 'high risk group – ? past infection?' *or* (if low risk or post immunisation check) 'immunity status check' on request form.
- Lab will test for surface *and* core antibody for the former, surface antibody only for the latter.

Results of blood tests (initial or post vaccine)
'Evidence of past or current infection' – get advice as to whether still active infection.

If active infection (HBS Ag positive):
- Give information about hepatitis B.
- Refer for specialist care.
- Consider management of contacts including testing and immunisation.

Immunisation not needed for antibody HBS *and/or* HBC positive (naturally immune).

HBS Ab < 10 IU

- Not immune.
- Full course of vaccine (even if this is second full course). If had two full courses, consider a non-responder, and reinforce advice about prevention.
- Another cause for non-response is current infection: check blood for Hb SAg
- Recheck six weeks after last injection.

HBS Ab 10-99 IU

- Need booster, recheck six weeks after this.
- If had booster give further booster to maximum of two, recheck after four weeks. If remain at 10-99 IU then re-boost at two years.

HBS Ab >100 IU

- Fully immune.
- Boost in five years.

Immunisation

- Immunisation given at nought, one and six months.
- Accelerated course (for example, for travel advice, but presented late) can be given at: nought, one week, three weeks and 12 months (or for those who have been exposed, see below).
- Record each dose on computer.
- Arrange follow up for next injection/post immunisation blood test at 4/52.

Post immunisation

- Check HBS Ab level 6/52 post immunisation.
- Re-immunise as per titre level (see above).

Hepatitis B post-exposure procedure for the non-immunised, or those of unknown current immunity

We may see patients who could have been exposed to hepatitis B through needle stick injury or unprotected sex with a known carrier of hepatitis B. The patient should attend for treatment as soon as possible after exposure to hepatitis B, preferably within 48 hours (but we can act up to seven days).

At first attendance
Record time of exposure, and what is known about source.

Blood test
- Take blood sample in appropriate tube for your lab.
- Label form 'Exposure to hepatitis B on (date), check immune status'.

Immunisation
- Give first hepatitis B immunisation.
- Contact local on call virologist to check if patient suitable for immunoglobulin and how to obtain this.
- Arrange time to give immunoglobulin.
- Arrange appointment for second hepatitis B immunisation.

Follow-up
- Hepatitis B immunisations to be given at one month, two months and 12 months.
- Blood samples to be taken at three months and six months, to check for infection.
- Blood sample to be taken six weeks after last immunisation to check immunity level.

Acknowledgements

We would like to thank Dr Sue Drake for her helpful comments on this chapter, and Dr Husam Osman for his assistance with the hepatitis B guidance.

Chapter 7

THE DIAGNOSIS OF HIV IN A PRIMARY CARE SETTING

Philippa Matthews

INTRODUCTION

Undiagnosed HIV infection is much more likely to jeopardise health or life. Currently around a third of HIV infected people in the UK are undiagnosed, and primary care can certainly play a part in improving this situation. There is evidence that undiagnosed patients with HIV-related symptoms are consulting in primary care, but their infection may remain undetected[1,2].

This chapter starts with a brief overview of the virus and its treatment, with references for readers who wish to explore these topics in more depth. Given the space available, priority has been given to HIV diagnosis and testing. Readers are referred elsewhere for more detailed information on HIV that is relevant to primary care[3].

EPIDEMIOLOGY

The HIV epidemic in the UK is currently growing at a fast rate. The increase in numbers of people accessing HIV care between 2003 and 2004 was 14 per cent. The total is now over 40,000. More than half are resident in London.

Practitioners should be aware of the patterns of HIV infection in the communities they serve. The international picture is important in helping to anticipate changes in the UK epidemic. Sub-Saharan Africa has the highest rates of HIV, but emerging epidemics in the Indian subcontinent and also the Caribbean islands are already having an impact on the UK picture because of close ties between our own population and these areas. Men who have sex with men also continue to be at higher risk as a group. Injecting drug users account for a small proportion of the UK epidemic to date (although the proportion is much larger in Scotland and in many other European countries).

Detailed and up-to-date epidemiological data is available from the Health Protection Agency website[4].

THE VIRUS

HIV is a retrovirus that is particularly characterised by its rapid mutation, leading to difficulties in both treatment and vaccine development. It is transmitted by exchange of body fluids, notably blood, semen, breast milk and also saliva. Transmission is aided by any breaks in the skin or mucosa, and several sexually transmissible infections (STIs) are associated with an increased risk of sexual transmission of HIV. Unprotected oral sex carries a real risk of transmission, although less than unprotected vaginal or anal intercourse. Transmission also occurs vertically (from mother to baby) at the time of birth and through breast-feeding.

THE NATURAL HISTORY OF HIV INFECTION

HIV preferentially infects white cells called CD4 cells, also known as T helper cells. HIV impairs the immune response (immunosuppression) because the number of CD4 cells falls as they become damaged and die. In the early weeks of infection the individual may experience a flu-like illness (primary HIV infection) and occasionally they may experience a short sharp drop in numbers of CD4 cells, with transient immunosuppression until the CD4 count recovers (see Figure 7.1, page 189). Thereafter, viral replication and the death of CD4 cells carry on for several years, but with a 'steady state' as lost CD4 cells are replaced. During this time the infected individual is essentially well. Ultimately, levels of CD4 cells can no longer be maintained. As the CD4 count declines, the patient becomes susceptible to infection and to some tumours. The amount of virus in the blood starts to rise and a measure of this (the viral load) is another useful clinical indicator. Physical problems caused by HIV itself also emerge.

COMMONER TERMS AND TESTS USED

CD4 count

This is a useful indicator of immunosuppression. CD4 counts of over 500 cells/μl indicate normal immunity. Between 500 and 200 cells/μl there is an increased risk of TB and a slight increased risk of some HIV-related tumours. Risks in this range are worse if the CD4 count is dropping very rapidly. Under 200 cells/μl, immunosuppression is profound.

Viral load
The viral load is a measure of the amount of HIV in the blood. If it is high, then the infection is not under control. A falling or undetectable amount of virus indicates that antiretrovirals are working.

Opportunistic infection
These infections are caused by organisms that are not usually pathogenic in humans with intact immunity. Immunosuppression is also associated with an increase in the incidence and severity of infections caused by well-recognised organisms.

Figure 7.1:
Association between virological, immunological and clinical events and time course for HIV infection

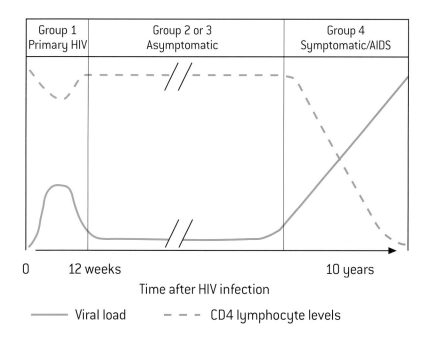

Reproduced with kind permission from ABC of AIDS (ed M Adler) from 'Natural history and management of early HIV infection' by A Mindel and M Tenant-Flowers (Blackwell Publishing, 5th ed, 2001).

Acquired Immune Deficiency Syndrome (AIDS)

This syndrome was defined before its causative virus (HIV) was identified. AIDS can be diagnosed if a patient has had one or more of a list of AIDS-defining conditions. It was, for a time, recognised as a mark of severity in HIV disease – a line crossed. The term is now much less commonly used, for two reasons. Firstly, there are much better means of measuring disease severity in individual patients (the CD4 count and the viral load). Secondly, thanks to antiretroviral therapy, patients who once had AIDS may now be extremely well, and their AIDS diagnosis is no longer relevant to them. AIDS remains a term used for epidemiological reasons, although epidemiologists are shifting to measures based on CD4 counts (as measured at diagnosis, to monitor late diagnosis of HIV, for example). AIDS remains a useful term where health care is poorly resourced. I do not use the term AIDS again in this chapter.

Window period

This is the time it takes for a person infected with HIV to become HIV antibody positive. For practical purposes it is taken as 12 weeks, although many people will have become antibody positive by four to eight weeks of infection. See P24 antigen test below, and see also HIV testing in primary care, page 200.

P24 antigen test

This test is indicated when the patient may still be in the window period (see above). As the name implies, it detects an antigen in the blood sample that is specific to HIV, although it may not be detectable until two weeks after infection. Increasingly laboratories are adopting HIV tests that combine antigen and antibody detection so that the window period is shortened compared to antibody tests alone.

Antiretroviral therapy (ART)

Antiretroviral therapy (ART) has been dramatically effective in saving lives in those countries that have been able to ensure consistent access to the medication. At least three drugs are used with each patient in order to minimise the chance for the virus to mutate and develop resistance. It is crucial for patients to take the medication regularly, because any missed doses benefit strains of HIV that are comparatively resistant and the benefit of a particular drug combination may be undermined. ART is started when there is evidence that the immunity of the patient has declined, and so patients with HIV may not be on treatment for some years if the infection is diagnosed early. In the early stages of initiation – or change in – ART, the viral load will give a good indication of effectiveness.

See Looking after people with HIV, page 204 for information on caring for patients on ART.

PREVENTION

Prevention of HIV transmission is attempted by a number of means:

- promotion of safer sexual practices, including condom use (with lubricant for anal intercourse)
- antenatal screening for HIV and interventions to prevent mother to baby transmission (primarily ART for both parties and avoidance of breastfeeding)
- treatment with ART following exposure to HIV, such as a high risk needle-stick injury ('post-exposure prophylaxis' or PEP). Practices should ensure that they have an emergency procedure in place, including a contact number, for dealing with needle-stick injuries. If indicated, PEP must be given as fast as possible
- work with injecting drug users, including anonymous needle exchanges, information on safer injecting practices and strategies to help cessation of injecting.

Attempts to improve diagnosis and treatment of STIs will, if effective, help to reduce the transmissibility of HIV. See also Further information, page 207.

Primary care has a part to play in most of these aspects of HIV prevention.

IMPROVING THE DETECTION OF HIV IN PRIMARY CARE

There are significant benefits if an HIV-infected patient is detected early:

- earlier diagnosis allows for monitoring and the commencement of ART, and also prophylactic medication before the patient becomes unwell
- there is better opportunity to prevent the onward spread of HIV if an individual is aware of their status
- there may be opportunities for the earlier diagnosis of others infected with HIV through partner notification
- the undiagnosed patient with advanced immunosuppression may be overwhelmed by a debilitating or even life-threatening illness before ART can be instituted or take effect.

Increased detection of HIV in primary care will depend on two things:

- improved recognition of the symptomatic patient

- increased HIV testing in asymptomatic people.

These will be discussed in turn.

The symptomatic patient

Broadly speaking, symptoms in undiagnosed HIV can be divided into two groups:

- symptoms and signs associated with primary HIV infection (seroconversion)
- symptoms and conditions associated with immunosuppression.

Once a patient is diagnosed and treated for HIV, a third group of symptoms – those associated with ART – comes into play. These will not be addressed here.

HIV has taken the place of syphilis as 'the great imitator'. One particular difficulty for the GP in diagnosing HIV is its tendency to present with common symptoms and conditions that have not in the past signified anything other than minor, often self-limiting, illness. In other words, HIV is the wolf in sheep's clothing. Of all the patients we see with a backache or headache, we know that very occasionally one may have a rare serious underlying condition that should not be missed. With HIV disease, a whole new array of conditions now need to come with the tag 'be careful not to miss . . .'. To further complicate the situation, our patient with a headache (who had a brain tumour) or with backache (who had spinal metastases) will get worse and return, whereas our patient with immunosuppression may get better from the condition we treated – although their immunity continues to be eroded.

Communication

The information about clinical diagnosis in HIV covered in this chapter cannot be divorced from the profound communication issues that arise. Raising the subject of HIV with a patient who is not expecting it may be very challenging for the clinician, and with the symptomatic patient this discomfort will usually be greater still. This chapter should therefore be read along with its partner, Chapter 2, which discusses strategies for both introducing the subject of HIV to the patient with symptoms and also doing a risk assessment for HIV. Learning about the symptomatic presentations of HIV, as covered here, is arguably the easy bit.

Primary HIV infection

The earliest opportunity that any clinician may have to diagnose HIV infection on the basis of symptoms is during primary HIV infection, also known as 'seroconversion illness'. Our first difficulty is that between 10 and 50 per cent of patients have either very mild symptoms or no symptoms at all when they are first infected with HIV. However the remainder represent our main chance to identify this infection early.

Primary HIV infection occurs up to ten weeks after infection with HIV. It is a flu- or glandular fever-like illness with a sore throat. The following conditions may also be present:

- myalgia, fatigue and sweats
- an associated blotchy rash, usually on the trunk
- oral, genital or peri-anal ulcers
- diarrhoea and meningism
- a transient immunosuppression leading to those associated conditions (for example, shingles – see Table 7.1, page 196).

If a GP is faced with a patient with a glandular fever-like illness, then they should try to allow the possibility of HIV to go through their mind. The clinical signs that would help distinguish this from glandular fever (the rash and ulcers, above) should be sought, but are not always present.

If primary HIV infection is a clinical possibility, then the subject should be raised with the patient and a risk assessment made. Then the GP and patient can have a discussion about whether to test for HIV. However, HIV antibody tests may still be negative at this stage, so it is *not* appropriate to do one of these in isolation. In the primary care context, a test for a specific HIV antigen (called P24) should be requested in addition, unless the laboratory already offers a dual test (antibody and antigen) as standard. Current advice is that the tests for viral RNA (viral load) on samples from primary care may not be reliable enough. HIV testing is discussed in HIV testing in primary care, page 200.

Some GPs feel that it is 'not fair' to 'raise worries' about HIV with patients with such common symptoms. Others feel that it is increasingly important to be ready to discuss HIV with patients – above all younger ones – in order to raise awareness of this preventable and yet increasingly common infection. In a patient with primary HIV infection, if the issue of HIV is not raised, then the patient will recover (this occasionally takes some weeks). A diagnostic opportunity has been lost, and their next presentation may be many years (and partners) later, when they have developed immunosuppression.

The immunosuppressed patient

The immunosuppressed patient is more likely to have:

- infections
- some tumours
- problems caused by HIV itself.

This section discusses the characteristic presentations of immunosuppression.

An approach to learning to recognise immunosuppression is to:

- familiarise yourself with the list of common conditions that are associated
- familiarise yourself with how pneumocystis carinii pneumonia (PCP) and other rarer, more HIV specific, conditions might present
- if you encounter such a presentation, then look for other clinical evidence of immunosuppression.

These steps will be dealt with in turn.

Common conditions and symptoms that are also associated with immunosuppression

Look out for these conditions, especially if:

- they are proving more severe or harder to treat than usual
- the patient has had more than one of them in the last two to three years.

Many examples of these conditions are listed in Table 7.1 (page 196). Try to remember the items in the 'condition' column so that you associate them with possible immunosuppression.

Rare conditions that are more specific to HIV

These are the conditions that the GP may not have seen before nor recognise, as they are so strongly associated with HIV. They are also listed in Table 7.1 (but in italics) according to which systems they affect.

Pneumocystis carinii pneumonia (PCP)

This is arguably the single most important 'new' condition that the GP should know about. This is because:

- it is life-threatening and the prognosis correlates strongly with how early the diagnosis was made
- it may have an insidious onset
- it presents at somewhat higher levels of immunity than most other very serious HIV-related conditions (that is, below a CD4 count of 200 cells/μl, as opposed to below 100 cells/μl).

The patient with PCP experiences respiratory symptoms that become progressively worse over a period of perhaps two to six weeks. They develop a dry cough and shortness of breath. Because of loss of elasticity in the lungs, they have a feeling that they are unable to take a full breath. They may or may not have a raised temperature. The patient might notice, for example, that three weeks ago they were very short of breath running for a bus, but now they notice it just walking. On auscultation the lungs may be clear and a chest X-ray may be normal. Apart from a chest infection, the GP may be thinking of asthma or even anxiety. If a GP encounters a patient with PCP, time may be lost if a chest X-ray is arranged or amoxicillin is given. The GP should consider whether there is other evidence of immunosuppression (see page 196), although PCP may be the first indicator of the problem. The GP can move on to discuss HIV with the patient. If PCP is a possibility, then the patient will need to be assessed in hospital and may need a bronchoscopy before the diagnosis can be confirmed.

Oral hairy leukoplakia

This condition is associated with EB virus, and causes white patches in the mouth – typically pale corrugations on the side of the tongue. It causes no pain or symptoms so it is not a helpful *presenting* condition. However it is pathognomonic of immunosuppression. Therefore the GP wondering whether a patient could be immunosuppressed should do a careful examination and look for this. Make sure you see pictures of it and examine the sides of a few 'normal' tongues to help you become confident about recognising it[5].

Kaposi's sarcoma

This is a tumour associated with a human herpes virus (HHV 8). It causes purple or dark brown indurated lumps in the mouth, skin, lungs, gut or elsewhere. It can become disseminated.

Cytomegalovirus retinitis

Cytomegalovirus (CMV) can infect the retina in immunosuppressed patients, causing blindness. However this only occurs at very low levels of immunity (CD4 counts of less than 100 cells/μl) and so this condition is very unlikely to be a *presenting* condition of immunosuppression. This is particularly good news for GPs, given that the patient with CMV retinitis will present with floaters. Incidentally, if you have a patient who you know to have HIV and who may have a very low CD4 count, do take care to seek advice if they develop floaters or other visual symptoms, as this infection is treatable.

Oesophageal candida

This condition presents with dysphagia and retrosternal pain and discomfort. It is highly likely to be associated with oral candida (although this is not guaranteed). Therefore the GP has a good chance of making the diagnosis *only* if they have a routine of examining the mouths of patients with dysphagia. Otherwise it may be diagnosed at endoscopy.

HOW DOES IMMUNOSUPPRESSION PRESENT?

Table 7.1:

Common conditions associated with immunosuppression and rare conditions that are more specific to HIV (see italics within table)

Affected system	Underlying cause	Condition	Comments
Skin	Viral infections	Shingles	Especially if multidermatomal or recurrent
		Molluscum	Especially in adults
		Herpes simplex	
		Warts	
	Fungal infections	Pityriasis versicolor	
	Bacterial infections	Folliculitis	
		Impetigo	
	Other/mixed origin	Seborrhoeic dermatitis	
		Psoriasis	May be very resistant to treatment
	Tumour (of viral origin)	*Kaposi's sarcoma*	*Purple or dark brown, indurated, sometimes bruise-like lesions. May cause a more generalised blotchy effect on eg lower limbs*

Affected system	Underlying cause	Condition	Comments
Mouth	Fungal infection	Candida	Florid oral thrush (except in small babies) should *always* lead to consideration of immunosuppression
	Bacterial infection	Gingivitis	
		Dental abscess	
	Viral infection	Aphthous ulcers	
	Tumour (of viral origin)	*Kaposi's sarcoma*	*Typically the hard palate, but may be elsewhere*
	Viral infection	*Oral hairy leukoplakia*	*Pale corrugations, typically on the side of the tongue (however is usually asymptomatic)*
Gut	Infective origin, including caused by HIV itself	Diarrhoea	
	Tumour (of viral origin)	*Anal intraepithelial neoplasia*	
	Fungal infection	*Oesophageal candida*	*Presents with dysphagia, association with oral candida likely*
Respiratory conditions	Bacterial infections	'Ordinary' chest infections	
		TB	HIV is now considered routinely with patients diagnosed as having TB
		Mycobacterium avium intracellulare MAI	*Atypical chest infection that occurs at very low CD4 counts (ie <100 cells/μl)*
	Tumour (of viral origin)	*Kaposi's sarcoma*	*May present with haemoptysis*
	Opportunistic infection	*Pneumocystis carinii pneumonia PCP*	*Progressive dry cough and breathlessness*

Affected system	Underlying cause	Condition	Comments
Systemic problems	Multiple causes, including HIV itself	Weight loss	
		Sweats	
		Fatigue	
		Anorexia	
Genital problems	Infective origin	Sexually transmissible infections	Consider in hard-to-treat warts and herpes. Remember risk association
	Fungal infection	Candida	
	Tumour (of viral origin)	Cervical smear abnormalities or cancer	Remember to consider the possibility of immunosuppression when referring for colposcopy
Nervous system	Multiple causes	Space occupying lesion	
	HIV	Peripheral neuropathy	
		HIV-related brain impairment	Associated with advanced, untreated HIV disease
Lymphatic system	HIV, other possible causes	Generalised lymphadenopathy	
	Tumour	Lymphoma	HIV is now considered routinely with (at least younger) patients diagnosed as having lymphoma
Eyes	*Viral infection*	*CMV retinitis*	*Floaters and progressive loss of sight*
FBC results		Neutropenia Anaemia Thrombocytopenia	*These abnormalities may be subtle, and a normal FBC does not rule out HIV*

Collecting additional evidence of immunosuppression

If a patient with a condition associated with immunosuppression is encountered
– perhaps they have hard-to-treat seborrhoeic dermatitis or a serious abnormality
on cervical screening – it is a helpful strategy to look for further evidence of
immunosuppression before the necessary step of raising the subject of HIV with the
patient. Here is a suggested approach.

Ask the patient if they have had:

- weight loss
- sweats
- diarrhoea.

Review the records to see if the patient has had any of the other conditions associated with immunosuppression in the last two to three years (for example, shingles six months ago).

Examine the patient for conditions associated with immunosuppression. Focus particularly on their:

- mouth
- skin
- nodes.

Consider which is more appropriate: An HIV test or admission? If a GP is considering that a patient may have PCP (whether or not there is other evidence of immunosuppression) then the next step is to ask for an urgent specialist opinion. With other diagnosed, or suspected, serious HIV-related conditions the course of action should be guided by the clinical state of the patient. If admission is the most appropriate option, then raising the subject of HIV with the patient at this stage may not be the priority, and will depend on how clearly the clinical picture points to HIV and how ill the patient is.

For most patients with evidence of immunosuppression, there is time for the GP to discuss and offer an HIV test so that they can be sure that any referral-on is appropriate. And so the subject of HIV – if it has not been raised already in the consultation – will have to be broached. Strategies for doing this are discussed in Chapter 2.

How to do an HIV test is discussed in HIV testing in primary care, page 200.

DETECTING HIV IN ASYMPTOMATIC PEOPLE

Increasing our ability in primary care to detect asymptomatic HIV infection depends upon both GPs and practice nurses:

- fully appreciating the clinical value of HIV detection (see page 191)
- being prepared to discuss HIV, risk of infection and testing when opportunities arise (see Chapter 2)

- having practice policies and templates that support and encourage discussion of sexual health and HIV with patients

- being prepared to offer and conduct HIV tests (see Barriers to testing below).

HIV TESTING IN PRIMARY CARE

Barriers to testing in primary care

Ready discussion, and availability, of HIV testing is undoubtedly necessary to reduce undiagnosed HIV. A system of HIV testing based on a specialised model (as was the case in the early years of the epidemic) necessarily leads to less readily available testing for patients. Already primary care accounts for almost a quarter of voluntary, confidential, HIV testing in Britain[6] (after the testing associated with antenatal screening and blood donation is excluded). Primary care has unmatched geographical spread and accessibility[7], and the National Strategy for HIV and Sexual Health[8] has recognised that HIV testing should be available in all practices.

There should now be no significant barriers to GPs and practice nurses using the HIV test – a basic clinical investigation – in primary care. We use other investigations which can diagnose a serious chronic illness, such as a glucose tolerance test, and we undertake other investigations that diagnose life-threatening illness, such as a chest X-ray. Finally, we deal with a range of conditions that have implications for the health of family members, for example, hereditary problems such as some breast cancers. However, HIV does still carry more stigma than many medical conditions; it may be that in the early days of HIV, this stigma affected even some clinicians, and thus their willingness to test. With the arrival of effective treatments – and antenatal screening for HIV – HIV is becoming more normalised and the stigma of testing is beginning to lessen. There remain some further barriers that will be discussed in turn, in the hope of dismantling them.

Medical reports for insurance purposes[9,10,11]
In the past, HIV testing has been treated differently to other investigations by insurance companies, because some companies discriminated against people who had had a test – even if it was negative. The argument went that these people represented a group at increased *future* risk of HIV. Things have moved on.

The Data Protection Act requires that *even if informed consent is given by the patient:*

- information released must be *relevant* and *necessary*

- information which is *excessive* should *not* be revealed.

If GPs use automatically produced computer reports generated for insurance purposes, each report must be individually edited to meet these obligations.

Guidance from the Association of British Insurers and British Medical Association[12] clarifies this requirement. GPs must not divulge information on:

- HIV testing – unless positive, or if the result is still awaited
- treated, resolved STIs
- lifestyle, including smoking, alcohol use, drug use, sexual behaviour or sexual orientation.

To support this guidance, there is an approved, standardised, form for insurance companies to use[13], for completion by GPs, although some companies may not comply with this. It is important that GPs are not drawn into completing non-compliant forms, as they may come in breach of the Data Protection Act. GPs may decide only to write reports for companies that use the approved form – indeed it may be simplest for GPs to insist on providing their own copy. By this means, GPs can avoid the need to check individual company forms for compliance.

Skills required for HIV testing

In the early years, when a positive result for HIV equated to a diagnosis for a terminal condition – coupled with the stigma and the implications for the health of partners and children – it could be argued with considerable reason that specialist counsellors were needed. With advances in treatment, the discussion of the test is much more straightforward, and the balance of benefits has shifted. Practice nurses and GPs with good communication skills already hold the skills needed to conduct HIV tests. A list of the issues that may need to be addressed with the patient is given later in the chapter.

Some clinicians may be fearful that they do not have the skills to be able to give a positive result. It is worth pointing out that there is time to arrange additional support (if needed) when a positive result is received from the lab – not least because a confirmatory (second) blood sample will be requested. These days, fear of detecting HIV should never inhibit a GP or practice nurse from offering the test to patients.

Time and resources

GPs and practice nurses should not over-estimate how much time it takes to conduct most HIV tests: in the majority of patients it will take ten minutes or less.

Once the clinical benefits of testing are clear to them, many GPs and practice nurses find they can incorporate this new test into their diagnostic armoury without difficulty (just as Helicobacter Pylori testing, 24 hour blood pressure monitoring and other investigations have become incorporated).

Giving a positive result may be time consuming, but for many clinicians this is rewarding – and likely to be only occasional – work. The second, confirmatory, sample that is required when a test is positive does give the clinician the opportunity to refer the patient on to a specialist clinic for this sample if they prefer.

Conducting an HIV test

The HIV antibody test may not become positive until up to 12 weeks after infection with the virus – this is called the window period. This delay to becoming antibody positive is perhaps the most important technical point about testing of which both the clinician and the patient need to be aware. However, now many laboratories have changed to incorporate a P24 antigen test along with HIV antibody tests, in which case they may detect HIV from as early as two weeks after infection.

If a laboratory only conducts antibody tests, then an antigen test (see P24 antigen test, page 190) can be requested if it is thought that the patient is still in the window period (for example when the patient may have primary HIV infection, see Primary HIV infection, page 192). Repeat antibody tests can always be arranged in three months if necessary.

What may need to be discussed with the patient:

Knowledge and understanding
- How HIV is transmitted, and risk to date.
- The benefits of knowing HIV status.
- What the test detects and the window period.
- Any need for a repeat test?
- Future risk reduction.

Implications for the patient if the test is positive
- How would the patient react?
- Family, partner, children, work, insurance.
- Coping with the wait for the result – does anyone know they are having a test?

Confidentiality

- A negative test will never be disclosed, but a positive one needs to be disclosed:
  - to health care workers outside the primary care team when relevant
  - when an application for insurance is made.

Consent

Practicalities

- Are there other tests to be done at the same time (for example, hepatitis B)?
- When will the patient get their result?
- Repeat test if needed?
- Check contact details.
- Give written information.

Giving results

The positive result

The laboratory is likely to phone with a positive result, asking for a confirmatory sample. In practice there is therefore a two stage process, and you will have time to get advice, written information and to clarify how to refer the patient on (and perhaps make an appointment). Remind yourself of what issues the patient had discussed with you prior to the test. The general principles of 'breaking bad news' hold for giving a positive HIV test, and will not be repeated here. However, the clinician should note that the prognosis is now much better than for many diagnoses we may make (although the patient may have a very stigmatised view). Point out the benefits to the patient's (and others') health of identifying the infection.

Issues of partner notification (informing sexual partners of risk, and the need for an HIV test) will be addressed through the specialist clinic. The GP with concerns about risks of infection to another of their patients should not disclose the risk of HIV but should first seek specialist — and possibly medico-legal — advice.

The negative result

There are two main points to address when giving a negative result:

- whether there is a need for a repeat test, due to the window period
- whether the patient understands how to protect themselves from HIV in the future.

In this chapter, priority has been given to improving the diagnosis of HIV by primary care: simply because of its life-saving potential. With respect to the care of people once they have been found to have HIV infection, the reader is referred elsewhere for more detailed information[14]. However, some of the more important practical issues that may arise are raised briefly here, in order to bring them to the attention of GPs and practice nurses and so they can seek further information.

The patient on antiretroviral therapy (ART)

Adherence

As the treatment is long term, it is extremely challenging for many patients to adhere rigidly to the treatment regimen. This is, however, of great importance to prevent the development of resistant strains of virus. The GP should not suggest patients stop ART without seeking specialist advice, which can always be sought on the phone if there are concerns about serious side effects. The GP or practice nurse may have opportunities to support patients in adhering to treatment.

Side effects

The side effects of ART are many and complex, and sometimes life-threatening. They may present with non-specific symptoms (such as lactic acidosis). One of the difficulties for the GP is that some side effects do not conform well to preconceptions about what is likely to be due to medication, for example peripheral neuropathy. It is well worth ensuring that HIV clinics update you routinely, and you keep a good record of the current medication, so that you can seek information if you are uncertain about side effects. Potentially serious side effects can be found in the BNF, and are also discussed in more detail elsewhere[15].

Interactions

Both drug and non-drug interactions can be a problem with ART, notably protease inhibitors (PIs) and non nucleoside reverse transcriptase inhibitors (NNRTIs). Substances from erythromycin to grapefruit juice are implicated, and interactions which decrease plasma concentrations of ART drugs may lead to problems with viral resistance (just as if the patient was missing doses). For detailed information see www.hiv-druginteractions.org (run by the University of Liverpool).

Notes on prevention and health promotion for the HIV-positive patient

Cervical screening

Women with HIV are at higher risk of cervical cancer. Cervical screening should be offered *annually*.

Immunisation

In general, live vaccines are avoided, but inactivated vaccines are safe. Guidance on immunisation of the HIV-infected patient, and also the baby born to the HIV-positive mother, should always be sought. The online (updated) version of the 'Green Book' can be found on www.dh.gov.uk under 'immunisation against infectious disease'.

Sexual health advice

Just as perfect adherence to ART is difficult, perfect adherence to safer sexual practices is also very difficult for most people. GPs and practice nurses should be prepared to discuss this and give what advice and support they can. Of all patients, people with HIV require ready access to free condoms (and, if required, lubricant). See Contraception, below. Even if both partners in a relationship have HIV, strains that are resistant to treatment can be passed from one person to another, and so the use of condoms (and lubrication) is still recommended.

Contraception

Drug interactions are a significant consideration in selecting contraception for women on ART. Information on the effects of individual antiretrovirals on plasma concentrations of orally taken steroids such as ethinyl estradiol (EE) and progestogens is still limited, and the effect of ART combinations is even harder to ascertain. It is possible that some sex steroids decrease the concentrations of some antiretrovirals, although (in an absence of appropriate studies) it is not thought that this is sufficient to lead to an increased risk of HIV drug resistance. In general, the efficacy of hormonal contraception taken orally, by patch or by implant is likely be affected by ART combinations (notably those including protease inhibitors and some NNRTIs), but it is not possible to advise women to what degree their risk of pregnancy will change. In general, these methods are therefore best avoided.

It is thought that both injectable progestogens and the intrauterine system can be used safely. There is no need for shortened intervals for injected DMPA.

IUDs and condoms are not affected – the latter are generally required alongside any other method of contraception in order to prevent the risk of infection of the partner (or the exchanging of resistant strains of virus).

If emergency contraception (EC) is required, a copper IUD is the method of choice for women on ART. If oral EC is to be used then the dose should be increased by 50 per cent, for example 2.25mgs of levonorgestrel, although there is no evidence for efficacy in this circumstance.

The evidence on the effects of drug interactions is being added to all the time, and so up-to-date advice must be sought. See www.hiv-druginteractions.org and the Faculty of Family Planning guidance[16].

International travel

Antimalarials may interact with ART. Further information on travel advice can be found elsewhere[17].

Key messages

- Primary care clinicians can play an important part in improving the diagnosis of HIV infection in the UK.
- Including a discussion of HIV testing as a routine part of sexual health care improves the uptake of testing.
- Progression to immunosuppression in those with HIV infection is largely preventable with antiretroviral therapy.
- The primary health care team can provide useful care, support and advice for those with HIV infection.

Acknowledgements

Many thanks to Dr Paul Thornton for detailed information and advice on current guidance and law relating to medical reports for insurance purposes.

Thanks to Dr Sue Drake for her helpful comments.

References

1. Madge S et al. Access to medical care one year prior to diagnosis in 100 HIV-positive women. *Family Practice*, vol 14, no 3, 1997, pp255–57.

2. 2. BHIVA audit. http://www.bhiva.org

3. Madge S et al. *HIV in Primary Care*. London: Medical Foundation for AIDS and Sexual Health 2004. Available at http://www.medfash.org.uk

4. http://www.hpa.org.uk

5. See note 3 above.

6. McGarrigle C et al. Investigating the relationship between HIV testing and risk behaviour in Britain: National Survey of Sexual Attitudes and Lifestyles 2000 *AIDS*, vol 19, no 1, 2005, pp77–84.

7. Audit Commission. *A Focus on General Practice in England*. London: Audit Commission 2002.

8. Department of Health. *National Strategy for Sexual Health and HIV*. London: Department of Health 2001.

9. British Medical Association (BMA). *Good Practice Guidelines on completion of GP Reports from the Joint GP IT Committee*. Available at http://www.bma.org.uk/ap.nsf/content/goodpracgpreports0804

10. Association of British Insurers and BMA. *Medical Information and Insurance. Joint Guidelines from the British Medical Association and the Association of British Insurers*. Available at http://www.abi.org.uk/display/file/child/106/blue_book.pdf

11. BMA and Association of British Insurers. *General Practitioner's Report (GPR)*. London: BMA 2003. Available at http://www.bma.org.uk/ap.nsf/Content/GPR

12. See notes 9–11 above.

13. See note 10 above.

14. See note 3 above.

15. See note 3 above.

16. Faculty of Family Planning and Reproductive Health Care Guidance (April 2005) Drug interactions with hormonal contraception. *Journal of Family Planning and Reproductive Health Care*, vol 31, no 2, 2005, pp139–51.

17. See note 3 above.

Further information

The following **fpa** leaflets may be useful for patients:

- *Your sexual health – where to go for help and advice*
- *HIV*

Available from **fpa**

Tel: 0845 122 8600
Fax: 0845 123 2349
Email: fpadirect@fpa.org.uk
www.fpa.org.uk

See also *HIV in Primary Care. An Essential Guide to HIV for GPs, Practice Nurses and Other Members of the Primary Healthcare Team.*
Available from www.medfash.org.uk

Chapter 8

SEXUAL DYSFUNCTION IN PRIMARY CARE

Gill Wakley

INTRODUCTION

The prevalence of sexual problems in the general population has been investigated by a number of community studies[1]. One study of several general practices found that 44 per cent of men and 36 per cent of women had sexual problems[2]. This and other studies show that GPs usually only record a diagnosis of sexual dysfunction in 3–4 per cent of their patients[3]. As health professionals in primary care, we need to become more aware of the overlap between sexual dysfunction and the mental or physical ill health affecting large numbers of our patients[4].

Proactive enquiry will help to prevent avoidable errors:

- If you miss sexual dysfunction, you will give the wrong advice or treatment, for example, investigating a couple who want a baby without realising that they do not have sexual intercourse.

- Your patients may not take important treatment, for example, medication for hypertension or depression.

- Unnecessary treatment can be avoided by understanding why patients present with somatic symptoms when they do.

- Recognising the importance of preventing sexually transmissible infections (STIs) such as chlamydia should help to make us proactive in asking about sexual behaviour.

Table 8.2 (page 224) provides guidance on common medical problems that lead to sexual dysfunction.

The consultation

Sexual activity can be difficult to talk about. It is usually a private concern, often alluded to by innuendo and non-verbal signals. Any discussions about sex and sexual difficulties may be accompanied by reticence and embarrassment on the part of the patient or the health professional[5, 6]. However, appropriate consultation skills can be used successfully to prompt a discussion. (See Consultation skills for sexual problems, below, and Chapter 2).

Consultation skills for sexual problems

- Use 'how the patient makes the doctor or nurse feel' to illustrate or interpret how the patient may relate to others[7].
- Notice and interpret non-verbal communication[8].
- Tolerate not knowing what to do – the patient has a unique need, so do not impose a solution from your previous experience but work with the patient to find the best solution.
- Recognise your own biases and prejudices.
- Have some knowledge of sexual functioning and emotional development[9].
- Use the physical examination as an exploration of emotional and physical factors[10].
- Give advice or reassurance only when you have checked that you understand what the problem is for the patient.
- Recognise when to refer elsewhere or suggest other avenues of help.
- Limit offers of help when the patient is not making progress.

If you ask a lot of questions you get a lot of answers – but you may not hear what the problem is because you have not allowed the patient to tell you. Health professionals need to study the emotional, physical and social aspects of a patient in order to understand how the whole person functions. Patients often have the information within themselves to enable them to resolve their sexual problems in the way that suits them best. You do not need to be an expert at sexual problems, just an expert at helping patients to find the solution.

Health professionals are very privileged to be able to look at the bodies of their patients. Listen and observe during the physical examination; it is not *just* to find or exclude physical abnormalities. The vulnerability of patients during physical examination often enables them to make connections between the complaint and the feelings. Offering to examine a patient can be very helpful. Notice if you are avoiding a physical examination and consider who, the patient or you, is afraid of what? Always offer a chaperone and respect the patient's wishes. Explain exactly what you are doing during the examination. The patient should be quite clear about the normality or otherwise of the examination as you proceed and understand why you are doing each part. Examining the prostate or inspecting the vulva may be obvious steps to you – but can be misunderstood by a patient unless you communicate the reasons and the findings in the context of the problem.

TYPES OF SEXUAL DYSFUNCTION

Sexual dysfunction may be:

- discovered as part of an on-going illness, as a side effect of treatment, or the result of disability
- presented openly
- presented after the patient has tried you out with a related (or even unrelated) complaint
- hidden by a psychosomatic complaint[11].

Illness or treatment affecting sexuality

Loss of interest in sexual activity while ill is common (see Table 8.1, page 215). The results of long-term illness can be divided into three parts – but each has its effect on the other.

The psychological effects of being ill

Individuals may feel sexually unattractive, embarrassed by how they look, or that they are not worth bothering about. Relationships change – a man or woman previously active and independent becomes reliant on others. Sex seems inappropriate, or even wrong, in this child-adult relationship. The couple may feel that sexual activity may damage the sufferer, or that the excitement of orgasm will be harmful.

The physical effects of being ill

Nerve or blood vessel damage directly affects the genitals, other erogenous zones or hormone levels. Pain, loss of flexibility and mobility, being too fat or too thin, all make sexual activity difficult or so painful that it is avoided even if desire is present.

The effect of treatment

Drugs may make the sufferer drowsy, depressed or too tired to bother, or cause direct effects on the erection or the orgasm. Surgery may damage the genital organs or remove part of the body that is felt to be necessary to sexual activity. Chemotherapy or radiotherapy can make the skin exquisitely tender and painful to touch. Treatment can also result in scarring or disfigurement, leading to loss of self-esteem.

COMMON PROBLEMS

Table 8.2 (page 224) gives information on common medical problems leading to sexual dysfunction.

Painful sex in women

- Without sexual arousal, deep pain from impact on the tissues can occur. The ballooning of the vagina and pulling up of the uterus will not occur without sexual arousal.

- Vaginismus can be secondary to dyspareunia or present as a phobic state preventing penetration. On rare occasions, the hymen is thick and tough, which can prevent penetration.

- Lack of lubrication following delivery, while breastfeeding or after the menopause, causes painful intercourse unless supplementary lubrication is used.

- Female genital mutilation involves procedures that include the partial or total removal of the external female genital organs. The extent of genital cutting and stitching varies considerably from country to country. The psychological and physical damage cause profound difficulties with penetrative intercourse but may be hidden because of fear of discovery or shame.

- Vulvovaginitis will cause pain, and the vaginal walls are tender and less well lubricated during the recovery from an infection or injury.

- Vulvodynia or vestibulitis result in superficial dyspareunia. Many doctors are unaware that these conditions exist. The pain around the opening to the vagina can be unprovoked, intermittent or prolonged, or only occur with attempted penetration. It may be localised to the vestibule, or affect other areas of the vulva and/or lower vagina. The appearance can vary from a bright red patch to looking completely normal[12, 13].

- Pelvic infection or endometriosis may cause pain on deep thrusting.

- A tender or distended bowel, common in conditions such as the irritable bowel syndrome or diverticular disease, can inhibit responsiveness.

- Constant pelvic pain which persists after negative investigations may be linked to changes in blood flow to the pelvic organs, which may in turn be affected by hormonal changes and psychological difficulties.

Painful sex in men

- Small tears in the frenulum can be extremely painful. Wearing a condom for a while after the tear has healed helps to prevent it happening again.
- Retraction of a tight foreskin with an erection may be painful.
- Infection or deformities of the penis can cause pain on intercourse.
- Sexual arousal not relieved by ejaculation sometimes leads to aching in the scrotum or the groin region.
- Small cysts in the epididymus can be tender when compressed, as well as often causing anxiety.
- Hernias or a hydrocoele cause mechanical difficulties and discomfort during intercourse.

Vaginal fantasies

Some women fear that intercourse will cause pain, damage or bleeding. Men also have fantasies about the vagina. These may prevent erection, cause loss of erection when approaching the vagina, or prevent ejaculation.

Fantasies have to emerge, sometimes at the time of examination, as they are not accessible by direct questioning. Never jump to conclusions about other people's fantasies on the basis of what you have heard from others, or what you might have experienced yourself. Clever theories prevent patients from explaining or exploring their own fantasies[14].

Sexual dysfunction following childbirth

Often patients date their sexual dysfunction to the birth of a baby. Remember that other changes may have been taking place at the same time – for example, moving house, separation or loss of parents, loss of job or status. Problems may have existed before, but were tolerated because of the desire for a baby, or an expectation that all would be solved by the birth.

For most couples during the course of a pregnancy, there is a reduction in the frequency of intercourse, and in interest and satisfaction with sexual activity. The couple may have anxieties about damaging the baby or triggering a miscarriage or labour. They may avoid, or feel guilty about, intercourse for these reasons. There is a wide variation between couples in sexual responsiveness, enjoyment and level of activity. Sexual problems after delivery are common, but few report discussing them with a health professional. One study showed that at three months, 58 per cent had experienced painful intercourse, 39 per cent vaginal dryness (this is especially likely if breastfeeding) and 44 per cent loss of sexual desire. Six months after delivery, 86 per cent had resumed intercourse. Yet, by eight to nine months after delivery, about a quarter to a third were still experiencing some problems [15].

Erectile dysfunction

Erectile dysfunction (ED) has been defined as the inability to achieve or maintain an erection sufficient for satisfactory sexual performance. ED is strongly related to age. While there is an estimated prevalence across all ages of about 10 per cent, the prevalence rises to over 50 per cent in men between 50 and 70 years, though it is not an inevitable consequence of normal ageing[16]. It is also associated with a number of organic disorders and diseases and is common in diabetes. ED may also occur with cardiovascular disorders (especially in men with angina or after myocardial infarction), neurological disorders, after pelvic surgery or trauma, and with pharmacological treatments of a number of diseases[17]. Although physical causes are common, remember that men will also have *feelings* of inadequacy and loss of manliness with *any* cause.

Responding to the complaint of erectile dysfunction

Take a sexual history to ensure that you and the patient are talking about the same condition. Many men refer to anything to do with sex as 'impotence', when the actual problem is ejaculatory. Find out when the difficulty started, if it is always present, or what makes it vary, for example, is it the situation or partner? Patients often want a physical examination.

Table 8.1:

Male examination

General inspection	Non-verbal clues about depression, anxiety, hypomania, etc.
	Distribution of facial and body hair or gynaecomastia for signs of endocrine abnormality.
	Breathlessness due to respiratory disease.
Cardiovascular	Blood pressure, peripheral pulses, other signs of arteriosclerosis or raised lipid levels.
Musculoskeletal	Difficulty getting undressed or climbing onto the couch may indicate problems with flexibility during intercourse.
Nervous system	If the history suggests a problem with the lumbosacral innervation check for sensation in the perineal or lower limbs.
Abdominal	Evidence of abdominal surgery, and the emotions expressed about it, may be relevant.
	Palpable bladder may indicate a prostate problem.
	Hernias can cause pain or obstruction to intercourse.
Genital	Note and discuss with the patient the appearance of the genitals.
	The size of the flaccid penis is very variable (5–10cm) and may seem smaller in obese men; many men think that their penis is 'too small'.
	Assess any thickened plaques if Peyronie's disease is suggested by a history of a bend in the erect penis.
	Ask the man to retract the foreskin, if present, and note any problems.
	Exclude any STI, for example warts.
	The testes should feel smooth and symmetrical; small epididymal cysts are common and can be tender; a varicocoele or a hernia may also produce tenderness above the testes.
Prostate	To assess for irregularity, asymmetry or hardness (suggestive of a malignancy) or tenderness (suggestive of prostatitis).
Rectal	For anal warts, haemorrhoids, or a fissure.

Investigations

Be guided by the history and examination. You would not consider doing a testosterone level in a young man who has sudden onset of erectile dysfunction after his girlfriend went off with his best friend!

Possible investigations include:

- testosterone level at 9am: low levels in the morning usually suggest hypogonadism in men

- serum hormone binding globulin to calculate the free androgen index (if available)

- luteinising hormone level: low levels suggests pituitary problem, a raised level suggests testicular failure

- prolactin level: raised levels may be iatrogenic, or indicate a pituitary problem. If only mildly raised, it may not be significant. The test should be repeated.

Other tests suggested by the history may include:

- thyroid hormone and thyroid stimulating hormone levels

- liver function tests (if drug or alcohol abuse is suspected)

- biochemical screen or full blood count (for example, in complaints of fatigue to exclude physical illness such as leukaemia or Addison's disease)

- prostate specific antigen if prostatic disease is suspected.

Treatment options

- **Changing lifestyles**: for example, reducing stress, giving up smoking, reducing alcohol consumption and taking up exercise may be all that is needed.

- **Changing prescription medication**: to one that does not have ED as a side effect.

- **Oral therapy**: several medications are now available including the phosphodiesterase type 5 inhibitors, sildenafil (Viagra), tadalafil (Cialis) and vardenafil (Levitra). Sublingual apomorphine (Uprima) appears rather less effective. They all require sexual stimulation as an aid to producing an erection. Men who are taking nitrates should not use phosphodiesterase type 5 inhibitors, or those who have a history of hypotension, stroke, myocardial infarction or severe hepatic impairment. Apomorphine is contraindicated in men who have a history of unstable angina, a recent myocardial infarction, hypotension or severe heart failure.

- **Hormone replacement**: to restore levels.

- **Counselling**: as ED can be caused and exacerbated by psychological causes, patients may benefit from counselling to alleviate anxiety, stress and reduce the effects on relationships. This is often used in conjunction with other treatments to enhance their effectiveness.

- **Vacuum devices**: some patients wish to avoid medication and can use an external vacuum device with one or more tension rings. The device is used to gain an erection by the use of a vacuum produced in a plastic cylinder and maintained by the rings at the base long enough for intercourse to take place.

- **Injection therapy**: the patient learns to self-inject medication into the side of the penis, which induces an erection that can last for several hours. The same medication (alprostadil) can be used in a pellet to insert into the urethra and the penis massaged to spread the medication into the tissues.

- **Penile prosthesis**: this involves an operation to insert a device into the two sides of the penis. The device can be either semi-rigid rods or an inflatable aid. A device should only be considered after all other methods have been tried.

- **Surgery**: occasionally the blood flow to the penis has been blocked either by injury or by vascular disease. Surgical removal of the blockage might allow erections to occur naturally.

Restrictions on NHS treatment for erectile dysfunction

Unless a man had been receiving treatment before 14 September 1998, only those in specified groups can be given treatment paid for by the NHS. These conditions are: diabetes, multiple sclerosis, Parkinson's disease, poliomyelitis, prostate cancer, prostatectomy including transurethral prostatectomy, radical pelvic surgery, renal failure treated by dialysis or transplant, severe pelvic injury, single gene neurological disease, spinal cord injury or spina bifida.

For other men who are caused severe distress by the condition, treatment should be available in exceptional circumstances after specialist assessment in a hospital[18].

Ejaculatory difficulties

Premature or retarded ejaculation can lead to patient and partner dissatisfaction with intercourse. A careful sexual history may reveal unrealistic expectations of simultaneous orgasm or comparisons with erotic fiction.

Treatment for premature ejaculation

- adjustment of the responsibility for success between the couple
- behavioural sensate focus techniques
- squeeze technique
- pelvic floor exercises
- clomiprimine[19] or a specific serotonin reuptake inhibitor two to three hours before intercourse (but beware those with intermittent impotence who will be worse)

- local anaesthetic (lignocaine spray) five to ten minutes before intercourse[20]
- using a condom, for example, Performa, to delay ejaculation.

Treatment for retarded ejaculation
- exploration of the power dynamics in the relationship
- exploration of the feelings of the man about intercourse and the vagina
- treatment of anxiety
- exploration of any fantasies that may be inhibitory.

Sexual violence

Child sexual abuse is the exploitation of anyone under the age of 16 for the sexual pleasure and gratification of the adult. It may be a single episode or continued over many years. It includes obscene phone calls or internet contact, voyeurism such as watching children undress, fondling, and taking pornographic pictures. It may include actual or attempted intercourse, rape, incest or prostitution. It represents a betrayal of trust (that adults will care for children) and an abuse of power (that adults will act in the best interests of children).

Despite the rationalisations put forward by the perpetrators, the effects are damaging and often persist long-term, especially if the abuse is repetitive over time and occurs within the close family (father or brother). Survivors of sexual abuse often blame themselves. They may harm themselves or feel constantly angry. They may have difficulty forming relationships and seek relief for their feelings through drugs, alcohol, food or unemotional sexual activity. They often have low self-esteem and may suffer repeated or long-term depression. The effects may be similar to post-traumatic stress disorder with flashbacks, distress and avoidance of male contact.

Many children who run away from home are the victims of abuse. People who have been abused may have such low self-esteem that they believe themselves worthless or only valued for sex. They are vulnerable to further exploitation as adults and may become prostitutes. Others are more resilient and may be able to put their experiences behind them.

Like child sexual abuse, adult sexual violence occurs in all walks of life and in all cultures. Most victims know their abuser and mostly it is a man abusing a woman. Some women may not have been subjected to any physical violence, but this does not make it any less terrifying.

Most of the information about the reaction to sexual violence is from women. Men tend to keep any episode of sexual violence more hidden. Some women will be able to struggle and scream; many become quiet and passive, especially if they have low self-esteem from previous abuse or lack of care. If they are from a culture where they have little power, they may feel unable to protest or resist. If they have been in a relationship where the partner is very dominant, again it may be difficult to resist. Women often feel guiltier if they have not been able to resist, as though they feel that somehow this signifies assent.

Afterwards the person assaulted has to cope with what has happened. He or she may be very tearful and distressed. However, we have all encountered people who cannot express how they feel either because of shock, or because not showing emotion is what they do in a crisis.

A sexual assault may make someone distressed for some time afterwards. They may find it impossible to allow someone else to touch them. Other people close to the victim may also need help and counselling. They may find it difficult to accept what has happened, blame the victim, or have problems with showing affection or love.

It is difficult to enquire about sexual violence unless it is volunteered. Direct questioning often results in denial. You need to build up trust before making open-ended enquiries that the patient can take up, if the time is right. In a recent article, only 1 per cent of women reported that they had ever been asked by their GP if they had been sexually assaulted. Almost one in five women objected to the idea of routine questioning on whether they had been raped or sexually assaulted. Significantly more women who had been forced to have sex reported that they would mind being asked by their GP if they had been sexually assaulted. This study showed that nearly one in four women reported experiencing sexual violence in adulthood[21].

Referral to useful organisations

The Rape Crisis Federation was established in 1996 to provide resources and facilities to support Rape Crisis Centres across the Wales and England. The federation acts as a referral service to women looking for help or support, putting them in touch with their nearest counselling service.

Mankind UK aims to support all men over the age of 17 years, through advice and help, who have suffered male sexual violence or sex attack, or have been sexually abused, sexually assaulted and/or raped, at any time in their life.

The Samaritans often provides support and advice for people in despair after sexual violence.

Domestic violence victims can also call The National Domestic Violence Helpline.

See Useful organisations, page 222 for further details.

Management and referral of sexual dysfunction

A skilled doctor or nurse can manage most sexual problems in general practice. Consider referral if the patient or couple want referral and:

- want to discuss the sexual dysfunction with someone not known to them
- have a problem that is beyond your competence
- have a problem that requires specialised or lengthy treatment not available in general practice.

Postgraduate training for non-specialists is available from courses organised by the Institute of Psychosexual Medicine[22] or approved by the British Association of Sexual & Relationship Therapists[23]. The Association of Psychosexual Nursing is also a useful resource[24]. Special interest groups of other organisations[25] and various universities offer courses and guidelines.

Patient information and support groups are useful resources both for professionals and patients. See Useful organisations, page 223.

Key messages

- As primary care practitioners, we need to become more aware of the overlap between sexual dysfunction and the mental or physical ill health affecting large numbers of our patients.
- While discussions about sex and sexual problems may lead to reticence and embarrassment for patients or health professionals, appropriate consultation skills can be used to prompt discussion.
- Patients often have the information within themselves to help them resolve their sexual problems. Work with the patient to find the best solution.
- Loss of interest in sex while ill is common, and may be due to the psychological or physical effects of being ill, or the effects of treatment.
- It is difficult to enquire about sexual violence unless it is volunteered. Build up trust before making open-ended enquiries that the patient can take up, if the time is right.

References

1. Dunn K et al. Systematic review of sexual problems: epidemiology and methodology. *Journal of Sex & Marital Therapy*, vol 28, no 5, 2002, pp399–422.

2. Dunn K, Croft P and Hackett G. Sexual problems: a study of prevalence and need for health care in the general population. *Family Practice,* vol 15, no 6, 1998, pp519–524.

3. Nazareth I, Boynton P and King M. Problems with sexual function in people attending London general practitioners: cross sectional study. *British Medical Journal,* volume 327, no 7412, 2003, pp423–426.

4. Watson P. Primary care and sex: too close for comfort? *Journal of Family Planning & Reproductive Health Care,* vol 29, no 2, 2003, p43.

5. Wakley G, Cunnion M and Chambers R. *Improving Sexual Health Advice*. Oxford: Radcliffe Medical Press 2003.

6. Thompson D. 'Disabled people aren't interested in sex . . .' (editorial) *Journal of Family Planning & Reproductive Health Care*, vol 29, no 3, 2003, pp125–126.

7. Balint M. *The Doctor, His Patient and the Illness*. London: Pitman 1964.

8. Neighbour R. *The Inner Consultation*. Petroc Press 1999.

9. Tomlinson J (ed). *ABC of Sexual Health*. London: BMJ Books 1999.

10. Skrine R. *Blocks and Freedoms in Sexual Life*. Oxford: Radcliffe Medical Press 1997.

11. Wakley G and Chambers R. *Sexual Health Matters in Primary Care*. Oxford: Radcliffe Medical Press 2002.

12. Stewart E and Spencer P. *The V Book*. Judy Piatkus London: 2002.

13. Patient information available from the self-help group htttp//:www.vulvalpainsociety.org

14. Valins L. *When a Woman's Body Says No to Sex: Understanding and Overcoming Vaginismus*. London: Penguin 1992.

15. Barrett G et al. Women's sexual health after childbirth. *British Journal of Obstetrics and Gynaecology,* vol 107, no 2, 2000, pp 186–195.

16. Feldman H, Goldstein I, Hatzichristou D et al. Impotence and its medical and psychosocial correlates: results of the Massachusetts Male Ageing Study. *Journal of Urology*; vol 151, 1994, pp54–61.

17. Hawton K. *Sexual Problems Associated with Physical Illness*. Oxford Textbook of Medicine (Weatherall D, Ledingham J and Warrell D, *eds*), Oxford University Press, 3rd edition, 1997, pp4243–7.

18. Joint Formulary Committee. *British National Formulary 46*. British Medical Association and Royal Pharmaceutical Society of Great Britain 2003.

19. Segraves R, Saren A and Segraves K et al. Clomipramine versus placebo in the treatment of premature ejaculation: a pilot study. *Journal of Sex & Marital Therapy*, vol 19, 1993, pp198–200.

20. Riley A. Premature ejaculation. *Journal of Sexual Health*, vol 4, no 3, 1994, pp69–71.

21. Coid J et al. Sexual violence against adult women primary care attenders in east London. *British Journal of General Practice,* vol 53, no 496, 2003, pp858–862.

22. The Institute of Psychosexual Medicine, 12 Chandos Street, London W1G 9DR or http://www.ipm.org.uk

23. British Association of Sexual & RelationshipTherapy, PO Box 13686, London SW20 92H or http://www.basrt.org.uk

24. The Association of Psychosexual Nursing, PO Box 2762, London W1A 5HQ or http://www.wanstead.park.btinternet.co.uk

25. British Association for Sexual Health and HIV (BASHH) at http://www.bashh.org

Further reading

Skrine R and Montford H (eds). *Psychosexual Medicine*. Arnold 2001.

Cooper E and Guillebaud J. *Sexuality and Disability – A Guide for Everyday Practice*. Radcliffe Medical Press 1999.

Wakley G and Chambers R. *Sexual Health Matters in Primary Care*. Radcliffe Medical Press 2002.

Wakley G, Cunnion M and Chambers R. *Improving Sexual Health Advice*. Radcliffe Medical Press 2003.

Useful organisations

Mankind UK

Mankind UK
PO Box 124
Newhaven BN9 9TQ
Tel: 01273 510447
Email: enquiries@mankinduk.co.uk
Website: www.mankinduk.co.uk
Offers advice and support to men who have suffered from sexual violence including sexual abuse.

National Domestic Violence Helpline

Helpline (24 hour freephone): 0808 2000 247
Website: www.refuge.org.uk
Information and help for women who are experiencing domestic violence.

Samaritans

Chris
PO Box 90 90
Stirling FK8 2SA
Helpline (24 hours): 08457 90 90 90
Email: jo@samaritans.org
Website: www.samaritans.org.uk
Can provide support and advice for people in despair after sexual violence.

Sexual Dysfunction Association

Windmill Place Business Centre
2–4 Windmill Lane
Southall UB2 4NJ
Helpline: 0870 7743571
Email: info@sda.uk.net
Website: www.impotence.org.uk

Rape Crisis

Email: info@rapecrisis.org.uk
Website: www.rapecrisis.co.uk
Gives details of rape crisis centres, and their helpline numbers, across the UK.

Relate

Helpline: 0845 456 1310 (Mon to Fri 9am–5pm)
Website: www.relate.org.uk
Offers counselling, psychosexual therapy and other services to help those experiencing difficulties in any adult couple relationship. Can give details of local centres, services and publications available.

Resolve – The Vaginismus Support Group

PO Box 820
London N10 3AW

Useful websites

www.brook.org.uk
Provides free and confidential sexual health advice and services specifically for young people under 25.

www.fpa.org.uk
Information about sexual health including online clinic finder showing details of nearest clinic.

www.impotence.org.uk
Information for men with erectile dysfunction, and their partners.

www.likeitis.org.uk
Information about all aspects of sex education and teenage life.

www.menshealthforum.org.uk
News, information, events and discussion on all aspects of men's health policy.

www.netdoctor.co.uk
Includes information on sex and relationships.

www.teenagehealthfreak.org
Health information for teenagers.

www.womensaid.org.uk
Information for women experiencing domestic violence.

Table 8.2:

Common medical problems leading to sexual dysfunction

	Problem	Possible solutions
Asthma	Fear of provoking an attack.	Use inhaler before intercourse.
Arthritis	Chronic pain and lack of mobility. Pelvic thrusting increases back pain.	Change established sexual positions. Adequate pain relief before activity.
Cardio-vascular	Either partner may have fears of death during intercourse. Angina. Impotence due to arterial damage, treatment, or psychological.	Information about the risks. Angina prophylaxis and avoidance of a large meal or excess alcohol beforehand. A more active role taken by the healthier partner.
Cervical smears and cancer of cervix	Self-blame or anger with partners. After treatment, may hear the *temporary* prohibition on intercourse as 'sex is bad'. Inelastic scar tissue may follow treatment. Fear of death or contamination of the partner.	Counselling and education. Avoidance of attitudes of blame. Careful choice of words and attitude during examinations and treatments to prevent the development of dysmorphic fantasies.

	Problem	Possible solutions
Colostomy or ileostomy	Adjustment to visible passage of urine or faeces. Orgasm can cause reflex filling of the bag. Pressure on scar or bag may be uncomfortable. Damage to nerves causing failure of erection.	Changing and taping flat the bag before intercourse. Changes in position, for example, the 'spoons position', to avoid pressure on the abdomen.
Contraception	Fear of failure. Removal of the risk can reduce excitement. Guilt or resentment. Alteration of cycle may be unwelcome. Barrier methods can be a barrier to intimacy.	Essential to match the method of contraception to the needs of the couple. An excellent method is no good if it is not used because it interferes with sexual function.
Diabetes	Loss of sensation or function. Impotence occurs in 35–59 per cent. Most women report no problems except those due to local vaginal changes or infections.	History, investigation and treatment should be available as for any other failure of function.
Hysterectomy	Altered sensation. Loss of lubrication during healing. The woman, or her partner, may fear the operation has made her too weak to withstand intercourse, or believe the woman is no longer feminine.	Counselling and information. Hormone replacement and/or lubricants. Removal of the cause of pain, excess bleeding, or discomfort may improve sexual function.
Learning disabilities	Often regarded as children with no sexuality. Limited sexual education. May be abused or exploited.	Sexual needs must be acknowledged. Privacy must be available. Appropriate sex education essential.
Mental illness	Loss of libido common in depression. Performance anxiety worsened by anxiety. Drug treatment may affect function. Dementia or mania can be accompanied by lack of inhibition.	Treatment of the underlying disorder. Change of treatment if function affected. Sexuality usually returns to pre-morbid condition after recovery.
Menopause	Myths about sexual activity in older people. Menopausal symptoms may inhibit sexual activity or cause discomfort.	Hormone replacement therapy may help the physical symptoms. Do not assume the cause is the menopause.
Prescribed medication	Side effects may cause sexual problems. Psychological reactions to illness or the need to take drug treatment.	Always ask open ended questions such as 'Have you noticed any difference in your sex life?'

	Problem	Possible solutions
Prolapse	Mechanical obstruction to penis. Bladder or rectum may empty.	Alteration of positions. Repair of prolapse.
Prostate enlargement	Finasteride may cause impotence. Surgery rarely causes impotence. Retrograde ejaculation after surgery is common.	Counselling and information. Alternative medical treatments such as alpha-blockers.
Recreational drugs	Difficult to separate the expectations from the effects. The high of a fix may be substituted for orgasm.	Address the psychological and interpersonal difficulties underlying the addictive behaviour.
Spinal injuries	Sexual desire is not usually affected. Bowel or bladder dysfunction. Spastic muscles. High spinal cord damage can cause a distressing condition in which sexual stimulation triggers headache, flushing and sweating.	Most people with spinal cord damage return to satisfying sexual activity despite considerable nerve damage. Pain and lack of mobility require alterations in technique and positions. The non-affected partner may need to become more active.
Strokes	Sexual desire usually seems to return to normal after 6–7 weeks unless psychological fears interfere. Occasionally understanding of when sexual activity is appropriate is altered and may cause offence. Physical disabilities. There is no evidence for the common fear that another stroke may be caused by sexual activity.	Counselling and education. Willingness to alter established patterns of positions, activity, etc makes resumption of sexual activity more likely.
STIs	Discomfort and pain. The stigma associated with infections. The feelings about the genitals, or about possible infidelity, can last long after the original infection.	Counselling and information. A non-judgemental attitude is essential. Acceptance of other people's sexual behaviour is important, while pointing out the dangers if necessary.
Phobias about STIs	The anxiety may have its basis in the prohibition of sexual thoughts or actions in childhood, or by religion.	Exploration of the inner fears and sexual prohibitions. Avoid repeated testing.

THE HANDBOOK OF SEXUAL HEALTH IN PRIMARY CARE

Chapter 9

SCREENING WELL PEOPLE

Muir Gray and Jennifer Hopwood

INTRODUCTION

This chapter explores the factors that need to be considered in delivering effective screening programmes. It looks at the criteria for developing programmes and considers different types of screening and the effects of screening on people who are well. The final section focuses on a number of issues relating to screening and sexual health.

All screening programmes do harm[1]; some do good as well. Debates about screening have been described as debates between snails and evangelists, with the evangelists keen to promote the benefits and the snails being aware of the harm that screening does. There is one other aspect of the harm that results from screening which needs to be taken into consideration, namely that some people who will be harmed by screening do not have the condition for which they are screened and which may be beneficially detected. Unlike clinical practice where people with a disease accept the risk of harm, in screening programmes some of the people who will be harmed stand no chance of obtaining benefit. The relationship between these two variables is shown in Figure 9.1 below.

The relationship between screening variables

	Harm from screening	
	No	Yes
Disease present — No	A	C
Disease present — Yes	B	D

The people in Group C are harmed but stand no chance of benefit.

The first step in policy-making is to determine which programmes do more good than harm at reasonable cost in terms of both health professionals' time and financial considerations. In deciding which programmes should be offered to the public, policy makers also have to take into account how research findings are reproduced in the ordinary service setting. Typically, a large research project covers only about one-hundredth of a national population and is carried out by dedicated professionals working to strict protocols. Hence it cannot be assumed that the level of quality, and therefore the levels of benefit and harm achieved in the research setting can be reproduced throughout the whole country.

As a result, policy makers need to consider the feasibility of delivering a programme the quality of which, while perhaps not matching that of research projects, is at least adequate. The relationship between quality, benefits and harms is shown in Figure 9.2 (page 229).

MAKING DECISIONS ABOUT SCREENING

There was tremendous enthusiasm for screening in the early 1960s. This was generated in part by the general uncritical enthusiasm for science, although this was to be brought low by the scandal of Thalidomide in the late 1960s. The early 1960s also saw the introduction of multiphasic biochemical testing which seemed to offer the opportunity for screening at low cost, at least at the point of testing. The situation was similar to the one in which we now find ourselves, with the ability to test for gene mutations in increasing numbers and at decreasing cost.

In the late 1960s there was a welcome surge of caution about screening with some important publications and the preparation of a report on screening by the World Health Organization. The criteria in that report, the so-called Wilson and Jungner criteria, have stood the test of time for 30 years (see Box 9.1, page 229).

Key factors in delivering a screening programme

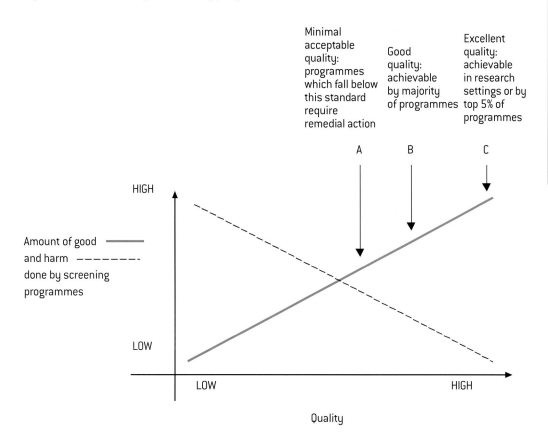

Box 9.1:

Criteria for appraising screening developed in the 1960s

- The condition sought should be an important health problem.
- There should be an accepted treatment for patients with recognised disease.
- Facilities for diagnosis and treatment should be available.
- There should be a recognisable latent or early symptomatic stage.
- There should be a suitable test or examination.
- The test should be acceptable to the population.
- The natural history of the condition, including development from latent to declared disease, should be adequately understood.
- There should be an agreed policy on whom to treat as patients.
- The cost of case-finding (including diagnosis and treatment of patients diagnosed) should be economically balanced in relation to possible expenditure on medical care as a whole.
- Case-finding should be a continuing process and not a 'once and for all' project.

When the National UK Screening Committee started work, however, it felt that the Wilson and Jungner criteria were weak in three respects:

- they did not put sufficient weight on the harmful effects of screening
- there was little consideration given to the strength of evidence that was put forward in support of a proposed new programme
- the opportunity costs of screening were not considered in detail.

For these reasons the National Screening Committee has developed a new set of criteria for screening to ensure that the Committee had good enough answers to the following questions:

- Do we understand the natural history of the disease?
- Is there a screening test of adequate sensitivity and specificity?
- Is there an effective treatment for the disorder?
- Is the programme as a whole acceptable to the population?

The criteria now used by the National Screening Committee are set out in Box 9.2, below.

Box 9.2:[2]

Criteria for appraising the viability, effectiveness and appropriateness of a screening programme – 2003

The condition

1. The condition should be an important health problem.
2. The epidemiology and natural history of the condition, including development from latent to declared disease, should be adequately understood and there should be a detectable risk factor, disease marker, latent period or early symptomatic stage.
3. All the cost-effective primary prevention interventions should have been implemented as far as practicable.

The test

4. There should be a simple, safe, precise and validated screening test.
5. The distribution of test values in the target population should be known and a suitable cut-off level defined and agreed.
6. The test should be acceptable to the population.
7. There should be an agreed policy on the further diagnostic investigation of individuals with a positive test result and on the choices available to those individuals.

The treatment

8. There should be an effective treatment or intervention for patients identified through early detection, with evidence of early treatment leading to better outcomes than late treatment.

9. There should be agreed evidence-based policies covering which individuals should be offered treatment and the appropriate treatment to be offered.

10. Clinical management of the condition and patient outcomes should be optimised in all health care providers prior to participation in a screening programme.

The screening programme

11. There should be evidence from high quality randomised controlled trials that the screening programme is effective in reducing mortality or morbidity.

    Where screening is aimed solely at providing information to allow the person being screened to make an 'informed choice' (for example, Down's syndrome, cystic fibrosis carrier screening), there must be evidence from high quality trials that the test accurately measures risk. The information that is provided about the test and its outcome must be of value and readily understood by the individual being screened.

12. There should be evidence that the complete screening programme (test, diagnostic procedures, treatment/intervention) is clinically, socially and ethically acceptable to health professionals and the public.

13. The benefit from the screening programme should outweigh the physical and psychological harm (caused by the test, diagnostic procedures and treatment).

14. The opportunity cost of the screening programme (including testing, diagnosis and treatment, administration, training and quality assurance) should be economically balanced in relation to expenditure on medical care as a whole (that is, value for money).

15. There should be a plan for managing and monitoring the screening programme and an agreed set of quality assurance standards.

16. Adequate staffing and facilities for testing, diagnosis, treatment and programme management should be available prior to the commencement of the screening programme.

17. All other options for managing the condition should have been considered (for example, improving treatment, providing other services), to ensure that no more cost effective intervention could be introduced or current interventions increased within the resources available.

18. Evidence-based information, explaining the consequences of testing, investigation and treatment, should be made available to potential participants to assist them in making an informed choice.

19. Public pressure for widening the eligibility criteria for reducing the screening interval, and for increasing the sensitivity of the testing process, should be anticipated. Decisions about these parameters should be scientifically justifiable to the public.

The case for screening is based on the assumption that most diseases follow the course set out in Figure 9.3, below. Screening may therefore aim to identify people at risk, or it may aim to identify people with asymptomatic disease.

Figure 9.3:

The course that most diseases follow

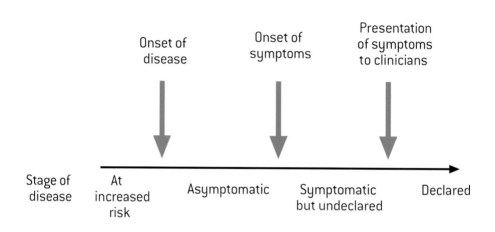

Screening for people at risk

The concept of risk is as difficult to define in screening as in clinical practice, but two main types of risk may be identified.

People at the end of the distribution curve

Everyone has a blood pressure, or cholesterol in their blood stream. However some have more than others, and there comes a point at which the individual has such a high level of blood pressure that the risks of treatment, not to be underestimated, can be accepted by the person and their clinician.

When identifying people 'at high risk', it is important to point out that this means they are at the end of a distribution curve. It is possible that only a minority of the people who eventually develop the disease may be detected, and a better result may be obtained by trying to shift the whole distribution curve. For example, if, through weight loss and exercise promotion, the mean blood pressure of the population as a whole could be reduced by 3 or 4 mmHg, then the effect might be as great as the effect on vascular disease that results from the detection of 'high blood pressure' and its reduction pharmacologically.

Individuals with a distinct risk factor

Some people are at risk because they have a particular disorder, for example familial hypercholesterolaemia. These people belong to a distinct sub-group of the population that can be identified and they can be offered treatment to prevent the disease.

Screening for disease

Screening for disease is apparently easier than screening for risk factors. The simplest model of disease would be a compound fracture and it is easy to distinguish between people who have a compound fracture and people who do not. However, the techniques used to distinguish between those who have a disease and those who do not are not so clear cut, and in clinical practice the same holds true. The ability of a screening test to discriminate between those who have a disease and those who do not is expressed as its sensitivity and specificity:

- the sensitivity of a screening test is measured by the proportion of people who actually have the disease that are picked up as positives by the test
- the specificity is measured by the proportion of people who do not have the disease and who have negative test results.

Those who test positive usually have to undergo a further procedure to reach the conclusive diagnosis. The constituent of elements of a screening programme are set out in Figure 9.4, page 234.

Elements of a screening programme

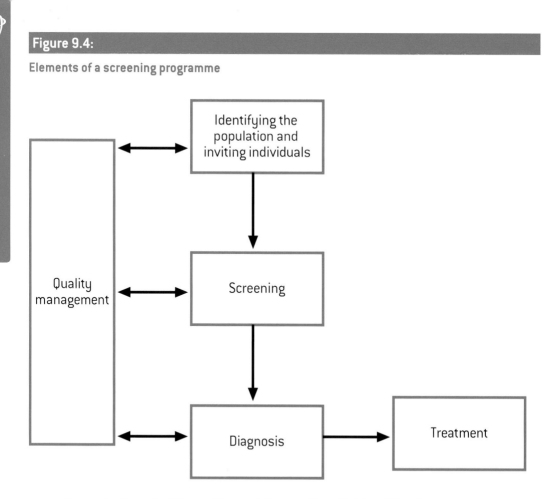

Screening is probabilistic; diagnosis is usually definitive. It is often remarked that one of the dramatic trends in medicine in the last 30 years has been the increased accuracy of diagnosis.

The grey zones of disease

Yet all is not clear cut. In some screening programmes, disorders are found where the significance is unclear. In breast cancer screening, for example, the significance of lobular and ductal carcinoma in situ remains a matter of debate. In programmes in which histopathology is used as the definitive diagnostic tool, the spectrum of appearances from obviously normal to obviously abnormal is continuous, with differences in expert opinion taking place in the grey zones in the middle.

In other screening programmes more cases are found by screening than would be expected on the basis of clinical data about the incidence of the disease, especially if the disease is asymptomatic or shows mild symptoms which may mask other conditions. In cystic fibrosis screening, for example, it is expected that more cases will be found as a result of screening than would be diagnosed clinically. Whether these additional 'mild' cases are significant is not known. One view is that these are people with chronic low-grade health problems who will benefit from diagnosis and treatment. Another view is that these people would have survived without any significant problems and will be disadvantaged by diagnosis and labelling. In screening for prostate cancer, some men found to have prostate cancer on biopsy will have surgical treatment resulting in incontinence or impotence with no assurance possible that the cancer that has been diagnosed by screening would have become manifest in their lifetime[3].

WHAT DOES SCREENING DO TO WELL PEOPLE?

All healthcare has adverse effects and a proportion of people are affected adversely by almost every intervention, even when given the highest quality of care[4]. There is, however, one hallmark that distinguishes the harm in screening – namely, the fact that some of the people who are harmed have no chance of receiving any benefit. In cancer screening, for example, a person who does not have colon cancer may have their colon perforated during the colonoscopy performed as a result of having a positive FOB test. This varies from one programme to another, depending upon the nature of the intervention, but because screening is offered to healthy people this dimension needs to be described in any information given to people offered screening. The adverse psychological effects of cervical screening are also clearly described[5].

In clinical practice, patients seek help. They need to know that the help they are offered may be harmful, but all the people who are harmed by treatment at least have the condition for which the treatment was intended. In screening, however, some of the people who suffer the adverse effects of screening do not have the disease that is the focus of screening, and therefore stand no opportunity of gaining any benefit.

Well persons

Patients, consumers or punters? In the debate about the status of people undergoing screening in Belfast, one side held that they should be called 'patients', the other that they should be called 'consumers'. One professional, however, said with directness and simplicity, "We just call them punters because, let's face it, they are taking a chance every time they come in". The term 'punter' is in fact a very accurate term to describe the person being offered screening.

Deciding who to screen

Within the whole population the first decision is to decide which sub-group within the population should be offered screening to maximise uptake. In chlamydia screening, for example, the decision was made to offer the test to women in the first instance. For abdominal aortic aneurysm, the decision is being considered to offer the test only to men. Such decisions are made on a combination of grounds of feasibility and practicability, together with cost-effectiveness.

Screens and sieves

The original meaning of the word *screen* in the seventeenth century was a sieve for sorting coal or grain or any other material. Depending upon the size and shape of the holes, this sieve was more or less effective. If the holes were too small, too high a proportion of the object that should have passed through was held back; if the holes were too big, many objects other than the desired objects could pass through. Somewhere in the twentieth century the word changed its meaning to indicate something that had no holes, as in a television screen or a screen in a lecture theatre.

The public have come to believe that screening should be 100 per cent sensitive and 100 per cent specific, an impossibility even in the best run programme. It is more appropriate to think of screening as risk reduction. All that can be offered is the possibility that the risk of death or disease will be reduced. If the limitations and adverse effects of screening are also spelled out then the person or punter can make a decision as to whether to accept the invitation or not.

Sensitivity and specificity

The screening test itself could be appraised with respect to various performance criteria, of which sensitivity and specificity are those most commonly used. The definition of these terms is set out below, together with a diagram showing their relationship.

- Sensitivity is the proportion of people with the disease who are identified as having it by a positive test result.

- Specificity is the proportion of people without the disease who are correctly reassured by a negative test result.

- A method for calculating the sensitivity and specificity of a diagnostic test is shown in Figure 9.5 below[6].

A method for calculating the sensitivity and specificity of a diagnostic test

	Disease		
		PRESENT	ABSENT
	POSITIVE	True Positive	False Positive
Test		A	B
		C	D
	NEGATIVE	False Negative	True Negative

On the basis of sensitivity and speciality of a test, the number of false positives and false negatives is calculated. However, the predictive value of a positive or negative test is a function not only of the performance of the test, but also of the prevalence of the condition in the population being screened.

SCREENING CONCEPTS

The term screening is sometimes used loosely to describe any check (history, examination or test) for a condition, but it may refer to an organised local or national screening programme. Programmes evolve in the light of evidence, for example, the age for invitation for cervical cytology, now starts at 25 years in England, instead of 20 years, and with three year early recall until 50 years, and then five yearly until 65 years.

Opportunistic case finding: at any consultation the subject is brought up and the test/examination offered there and then.

Opportunistic recruitment: it is mentioned at a consultation that screening is available, when and where, so that an appointment can be made for a future date.

Call/recall: everyone in a target age group or other category are invited at intervals, for example, the NHS Cervical Screening Programme (NHSCSP).

Targeted: certain populations, for example, antenatal syphilis serology; or groups of people at special risk, for example, pre-abortion chlamydia screening.

Mandated: screening is a condition of acceptance, for example, employer-initiated or for insurance.

Elective/self-initiated: in the private sector or requested, for example, in a department of genitourinary medicine (GUM) or general practice. Self-initiated testing may even be done by sending a sample via an internet advert and receiving the result to action.

SCREENING AND SEXUAL HEALTH

Some screening programmes impact indirectly on sexual health, such as those for breast or testicular cancer, cervical screening or prostate cancer screening. It is important for health professionals to recognise natural concerns.

Women attend health services – general practice and family planning clinics – for services such as contraception, antenatal care, abortion and immunisations for children. Therefore, they have traditionally been seen as more accessible targets than men for medically initiated screening programmes. Such screening includes syphilis serology and HIV testing in antenatal care; blood pressure monitoring in combined oral contraceptive takers; and the offer of a cervical smear opportunistically to those who are non-responders to their call/recall letter. A recent finding that 65 per cent of men attended their GP in the past year should enable us to facilitate the inclusion of men in screening. There are also innovative ways of facilitating access for both men and women, for example, chlamydia testing in pharmacies or email and web based services.

In the field of sexual health, as it relates to the prevention of tubal factor infertility (TFI) in women, there are several inconsistencies in healthcare delivery and these are perpetuated by differences in education, interest and funding. It is something of a lottery and depends on the health service consulted and the health professional seen, as to what is offered. Some examples of this are given below.

- Well woman/man clinics may offer different examinations and tests but not all offer chlamydia screening.
- Cervical smears may be used inappropriately; they should not be used to diagnose or exclude infections.
- Symptoms such as discharge, dysuria and abnormal bleeding may be attributed to candida, cystitis and hormone problems respectively, when in reality they may be due to chlamydial infection.
- Pelvic inflammatory disease (PID) may be treated but no reference is made to the partner(s) who may also need treatment if the woman risks reinfection.

- Furthermore, traditional diagnostic medicine does not address the fact that most chlamydial infection is asymptomatic, and so is overlooked.

To some extent these differences in practice can be avoided by participation by all services in a chlamydia screening programme for those in the target age group, and testing those of any age where there are relevant symptoms or risk factors. Sexual health networks can develop common care pathways and reduce such differences in approach.

Chlamydia screening

Considering chlamydia in relation to the parameters for screening:

- **The condition should be common and serious**: it is found in 10 per cent of young people who have ever had sex who are tested in health/non-health care settings. It is one cause of PID, which can lead to TFI, ectopic pregnancies and pre-term delivery.

- **There should be an asymptomatic stage**: at least 70 per cent of women and 50 per cent of men found to have chlamydia are asymptomatic.

- **The natural history should be known**: much is known but not all. There are likely to be both host and organism factors making some people more likely to suffer the sequelae. These may become clearer with time.

- **The programme should be acceptable**: using nucleic acid amplification tests (NAATs), the antigen is amplified so that the small amount which may be present in urine or a self-taken vulvo-vaginal swab can be detected, as well as the conventional swab sample which requires a clinical examination.

- **There should be a good test**: NAATs are sensitive and specific, but no test is 100 per cent accurate. This is important information to give to those taking the test.

- **Timely, evidence-based and effective management of screened positive people must exist**: use of the correct antibiotics for patient and partner(s), that is, azithromycin or doxycycline (or erythromycin if risk of pregnancy) are effective.

- **Harm should be minimised**: there is a risk of focusing solely on chlamydia. Reducing risk-taking, use of condoms, contraception, and other infections and conditions must not be forgotten. False reassurance, derived fron a negative result, could lead to a continuing risky lifestyle. Also, even if treated, women do worry about future fertility. There is the risk of blame and the ending of relationships, so it is essential to pre-empt this sensitivity in the light of the fact that infection may persist for some time from a previous relationship and that there can occasionally be false results.

Box 9.3:

The National Chlamydia Screening Programme in England

Phased implementation of a National Chlamydia Screening Programme (NCSP) in England began in 2003, with full national coverage in place by March 2007. The aim of the NCSP is to control chlamydia through early detection and treatment of those with asymptomatic infection; to reduce prevalence through effective partner notification and treatment; and to prevent the consequences of untreated infection. Opportunistic screening for chlamydia is offered to sexually active women and men under 25 years when they attend a range of healthcare settings or non-clinical screening venues.

The NCSP currently recommends young people are encouraged to get screened annually or whenever there is a change in sexual partners. A minimum of five weeks is needed between tests following a positive result. Repeat testing before this time may detect non-viable organisms from the previous infection. Management of partners is crucial to the success of the programme.

See www.dh.gov.uk and www.hpa.org.uk for further information.

If offering a chlamydia test opportunistically, it is easier if there is background information available so that it can simply be asked *"Are you up to date with . . . ?"* Computer support can be used to flag those in the target age range. The offer can be made by any member of the team – nurse, doctor, or staff at other sample collection sites, for example, colleges or pharmacies.

Local organisation and delivery of the NCSP can provide robust, fail-safe systems for tracking results, informing people of their results, arranging treatment, ensuring partners are contacted for testing and treatment and data reporting. Arrangements vary in different localities but should be sustainable and clearly understood by all health professionals and others engaged in screening. While in some areas the chlamydia screening office team manage the follow-up of those testing positive, in others, screening venues in general practice or community contraceptive services are now involved in treatment and partner notification. Community health advisers can also provide support.

Screening or diagnosis?

Chlamydia testing is an all inclusive term for every chlamydia test performed, regardless of reason for testing, setting or location where tested, type of test used or population tested. The term screening is used when people are tested despite not having symptoms and/or when people would have been unlikely to access such testing.

Confusion sometimes arises about whether to categorise chlamydia testing as 'diagnostic' or 'screening', for example, in those who accept the offer of a screen and only later volunteer symptoms. If they meet defined target criteria for the NCSP, and would not otherwise have sought testing or reported symptoms without the screening offer, their test can still be recorded as a screen. However, in addition to screening for chlamydia, the clinical management of such a person may need to include examination and diagnostic investigation of symptoms.

Definitions of diagnostic testing or screening are broad. The source of funding may vary depending upon whether testing is undertaken as part of a screening programme, for diagnostic testing or other routine screening, such as that which may be provided in advance of abortion. Chlamydia screening provided for women within the target age group prior to abortion may already be funded outside of the NCSP and it's important to clarify this, as well as who is responsible for treatment or data reporting.

Multidisciplinary collaboration and joined-up working at local level is crucial for the success of screening programmes. Local chlamydia screening teams are encouraged to collaborate with existing (and potential) providers of chlamydia testing to standardise care and clarify the extent and limits of screening programme responsibility.

A number of questions arise in a chlamydia screening programme:

- If a person is screened outside their general practice, should their results be sent to their GP as well as the test initiator, as in the cervical screening programme? The latest British Medical Association/Association of British Insurers guidelines state that management of uncomplicated episodes of sexually transmissible infection (STI), even a series of such, do not offer any bar or prejudice to insurance cover. Exact interpretation of these words in every case may be difficult and not reassure everyone.

- How often should screening be offered? The NCSP for under 25-year-old men and women recommends annual screening and at each partner change.

- How can we measure 'coverage' of a population? Should we link results from different practices/areas as in cervical cytology, or to other services, for example, GUM? Should there be medical record linkage?

- Are non-acceptors of tests at most risk or have they not had a sexual partner? It is important that those offering tests have the skills required to help people evaluate their risks, whether directly or in devising a self-evaluation form or interactive computer screen.

- Are there prescription charges for chlamydia treatment? Treatment for chlamydia within the NCSP is provided free of charge. local chlamydia screening offices will provide treatment supplies. Treatment for all STIs is free in GUM departments and many contraceptive clinics.

Key messages

- The first step in policy-making is to determine which programmes do more good than harm at reasonable cost in terms of both health professionals' time and financial considerations.
- Screening should be thought of in terms of risk reduction, rather than 100 per cent sensitive and 100 per cent specific. If the limitations and adverse effects are spelled out, then the person can make a decision about whether to accept the invitation or not.
- England has launched a major public health programme, the NCSP. Opportunistic screening for chlamydia is offered to young people in a locally determined set of clinical and non-clinical venues, supported in a national framework of practice guidelines in accordance with the agreed principles of ethical screening practice.

Acknowledgements

Many thanks to members of the NCSP management and advisory group (CAC) for their comments on this chapter.

References

1. Gøtzsche P C and Jorgensen K J. Model of outcomes of screening mammography; information needs to support informed choices. *BMJ*, vol 331, no 7512, 2005, pp 350–1.

2. Department of Health. Screening of pregnant women for hepatitis B and immunisation of babies at risk. *Health Service Circular: HSC 1998/127*. London: Department of Health, 1998. Wilson J M G and Jungner G. Principles and practice of screening for disease. *Public Health Paper Number 34*. Geneva: WHO, 1968. Cochrane A L and Holland W W. Validation of screening procedures. *British Medical Bulletin*, vol 27, 3–8, 1971. Sackett D L and Holland W W. Controversy in the detection of disease. *The Lancet,* vol 2, no 7930, 1975, pp357–9. Wald N J (Ed). *Antenatal and Neonatal Screening*. Oxford: Oxford University Press, 1984. Holland W W and Stewart S. *Screening in Healthcare*. London: The Nuffield Provincial Hospitals Trust, 1990. Gray J A M. *Dimensions and Definitions of Screening*. Milton Keynes: NHS Executive Anglia and Oxford, Research and Development Directorate, 1996.

3. Prostate Cancer Risk Management Programme Scientific Reference Group. Review of screening for prostate cancer. *BJU International*, vol 95, Supplement 3, April 2005.

4. Institute of Medicine. *Crossing the Quality Chasm: A New Health System for the 21st Century*. The National Academy Press, 2001.

5. Quilliam S. *Positive Smear*. Charles Letts & Co Ltd, 1992.

6. Gray J A M. *Evidence-Based Healthcare*. Churchill Livingstone, 2001.

Chapter 10

SEXUAL HEALTH – LEARNING FROM CONSUMERS

Toni Belfield

INTRODUCTION

Obtaining harmonised, objective information on reproductive and sexual health is not only a necessity; it is also a right. Such knowledge provides an understanding of how health, emotions and behaviours relate to fertility. It enables an unravelling of myths, misconceptions and misinformation. Importantly, it can minimise the embarrassment and anxiety that all too often surrounds this area of health. Good medical practice relates to mutual respect between the professional – an expert in the area of health care being discussed, and the individual – an expert about themselves. It must include good information-sharing and ideally high quality continuity of care. Knowledge provides empowerment and confidence, which in turn enables improved reproductive and sexual health decisions to be made.

Patients, consumers, users, clients are all terms for women and men who receive sexual health services. The reality is that whatever we call people who see us for information, advice, support or treatment – *without them we would have no role.* Recognising this is important – it is central to providing a service that knows and understands what people like or dislike and which addresses people's expectations, needs, worries and concerns. For this chapter, the term *consumers* is used for people who use or may wish to use sexual health services. There is no universal agreement about the words meant to specify people who use health care. However, people accessing sexual health services are generally 'well' people and as such should not be called patients who are seen in the context of ill health. This is not just semantics. How we refer to people in relation to health care services affects how we communicate and share knowledge, and has the potential to shift the balance of power between provider and user to one of shared discussion and decision.

Sexual health encompasses contraception, planning a pregnancy, issues around pregnancy choices, including abortion, screening, testing, treatment for sexually transmissible infections (STIs) and help with sexual dysfunction. Sexual health services may be delivered under 'one roof' or separately by providers in different settings. *Wherever* they are provided the pathways to different sexual health services for consumers need to be clear and seamless. The National Strategy for Sexual Health and HIV[1] sets out a framework for how sexual health services should be provided in England. Similar strategies are available in Wales, Scotland and Northern Ireland. Resources, 'tool kits' and standards are available to support and improve sexual health services and care[2,3,4,5]. These are useful and need to be known about, and also used.

In the many discussions of where sexual health should be provided, the unique role of general practice is important. Most people's first point of contact with the health care profession is with their GP. Unlike community clinic or hospital services that offer 'specialist' services, general practice offers a totally holistic health service, which should include sexual health. In general practice there is a different relationship between user and provider, women and men attend a practice for *all* their health needs. This enables ongoing therapeutic relationships to be established with the general practice team which can include advice, information, screening, testing and treatment for sexual health issues where necessary as part of general health care. In addition the diversity of the general practice team (see Chapter 1) provides women and men with choices about who to see depending on gender preferences or the specific health issue that requires help. In reality, general practice has the potential to offer the best 'one stop' shop for health. However, it is important to understand that both professionals and health care users find it difficult to address some areas of sexual health – embarrassment, 'opening cans of worms' which may disclose information, lack of expertise, and understanding or knowledge of how to raise sexual health concerns (see Chapter 2) are issues that affect both user and provider. In recognition of this, the information provided in this chapter looks at how sexual health issues are considered generally.

SEXUAL LIFESTYLES AND BEHAVIOUR

Sexual behaviours and attitudes are complex and their outcomes have wide practical implications. People are starting sexual activity earlier, have more sexual partners, use contraception more, but not consistently, and STIs and unplanned pregnancy are increasing. Findings from the National Survey of Attitudes and Lifestyles[6,7,8] illustrate that there is a wide variability in sexual lifestyles by age, gender, relationships and residence and that this is *normal.* Research continues to confirm that people do not always behave rationally or in an organised or planned manner with their sex lives, and people do and will take risks intentionally or unintentionally. Importantly, sexual lifestyles relate directly to factors such as knowledge and education, employment, deprivation and inequalities.

UNDERSTANDING CONSUMERS' VIEWS

As part of the NHS Plan to modernise services, public and patient user-involvement is now central to service development[9,10,11]. This involves consumers having a central role in how services are designed, developed and delivered in primary and secondary care. In general practice, the General Medical Services Contract (2004) incorporates national quality indicators (the Quality Outcomes Framework) addressing patient experience. Mechanisms must be put in place to ensure that all views are obtained from consumers, potential and past users of services, carers and people of all ages, sexual orientation, gender and abilities. Consumer and patient groups, guidance and advice is widely available to support this process[12,13,14,15].

How we consider issues to do with sex – how we talk about it and how we deliver services to support sexual wellbeing – has enormous impact on how services will be known about *and* used. Women and men's sexual health needs, expectations and choices are influenced by many factors: knowledge, information, lifestyle need, age, abilities, sexual orientation, religion, ethnicity, perceptions (their own *and* others), anxiety and embarrassment. A provider's preferences and assumptions about individuals and service delivery contributes greatly to limiting or improving acceptability and choice. Attempts to categorise people's needs simplistically such as age, parity or social class reflect neither the complexity of their lives, nor the many factors which influence sexual relationships and reproductive choices.

What do people want to know about services?

- What services are available? Where services are available? When are they available?
- How do I access services? What if I am unable to access services?
- Who will I see? Can I choose who to see?
- How will I be treated?
- Will it be confidential?

- What information will I be given?
- What choices will I have?
- What if I don't understand?
- How do I get more information if I need it?
- Can I bring anyone with me?
- How do I provide comment or feedback on the service I have received?

fpa helpline and information services handle over 100,000 enquiries annually from the public and professionals. These enquiries illustrate on a daily basis the difficulties that people have in knowing about and accessing good information on sexual health and about services. DIPEx (Database of Personal Experiences of Health and Illness) shows that although there is a wealth of information, it is a maze[16]. As such, people are unable to find what they need to know when they need it.

"It's mainly getting hold of information, that's the hardest thing – you're not sure where to go, especially if it is something you are embarrassed about." [17]

Much of the information we have on people's views of sexual health services relates to young people's views. Their messages are clear and consistent: they focus directly on the need for confidential services that are friendly and non-judgemental[18,19]. Young people's needs 'mirror' views, anxieties and needs of *all* ages and abilities which **fpa** hears everyday through its helpline services. These include:

- not wishing to be stereotyped, criticised or judged (*'foolish', 'feckless', 'promiscuous', 'irresponsible', 'too young', 'should know better'*)
- the wish to be treated 'properly', with respect
- to be listened to *and* understood – not interrogated
- to be given 'permission' to voice fears or anxieties
- to be given empathy with the situation
- to receive confidential services and *know* they are confidential
- to be given 'time'
- to be given more information.

In supporting younger people accessing services, specific guidance is available to support practice[20,21]. Burack's study[22] of 1,045 young people aged 13–15 showed that even among this age group, most were aware that general practice provided contraception and pregnancy testing services, smears and some condom provision.

However, over a quarter thought you had to be over 16 and many feared 'wasting' a GP's time. This 'fear' of wasting a professional's time about a sexual health concern is a common worry from women of all ages. Typical **fpa** helpline examples include:

- *"it's not really important"*
- *"I don't want to bother the doctor"*
- *"I am sure it (symptom) will go away"*
- *"could the pharmacist deal with this?"*
- *"will they mind if I go to see them?"*

Research shows that embarrassment and confidentiality are vitally important concerns for all women attending sexual health services. Work by Seamark and McPherson[23,24] also illustrates that finding out what women want, and being responsive to need, supports attendance, reassures women that consultations are confidential and shows that embarrassment at attending in general practice decreases with age, as well as the preference to see a female doctor.

While women are seen more within health care services, men are often invisible – yet sex and procreation take two! Health care needs vary between men and women, especially sexual and reproductive health concerns. Healthy women will frequently be involved in health care through cervical smears, breast awareness, contraceptive care or pregnancy, and such contact with health services may start at a very young age. Men have no similar 'start'[25]. Sexual health policies and services do not address men's needs and experiences well. The Men's Health Forum indicates that 'there is still too little understanding of the impact of gender on men and their sexuality and of the implications this has for tackling men's health problems'[26]. Where research does exist, information for men tends to relate to condom provision[27]. Services need to involve men and create an environment that addresses their needs and perspectives.

It is not just men whose needs are invisible or not understood. Disabled people still feel that their sexual health information and service needs are not well addressed, and that they are seen as:

'a separate category of people with no gender or sexuality, a category of people whom some health professionals and even our own families, do not consider capable of making basic decisions about our own sexuality, fertility, or sexual health: who don't need smears or mammograms.'[28]

Making such assumptions about people with physical or learning disabilities removes their rights to have the same choices and needs as those without disability and contributes to discrimination. For example, recognise the difficulties women with sight or hearing impairment may have in relation to taking a cervical smear, carrying out an STI test or discussing what an IUD looks like and how it is inserted.

Transcultural, religious and ethnic needs[29] are important to acknowledge and understand. For example, the importance of using the left or right hand in eastern cultures impacts directly on how condoms or diaphragms are used. Contraceptive methods that affect menstruation or bleeding patterns have specific implications for Sikh, Muslim or Jewish women where menstrual bleeding prevents certain religious duties and household tasks.

Older people, just like the young, have loving, passionate relationships which include sex. Yet, often this is not acknowledged by health professionals. They are often discouraged as a result of myth, societal stereotyping and negative attitudes[30]. Illness and sexuality is another taboo. DIPEx[31] illustrates that some areas such as sex are too uncomfortable to address:
'People who have cancer describe how sexual difficulties were ducked and how they struggled to maintain their persona.'

Equally, whether young or old, with or without disability, ill or healthy, sexual orientation is central to who and what we are. As such, sexual history-taking and questions require sensitive exploration, avoiding assumptions and prejudice (see Chapter 2). Widespread homophobia and heterosexism still exist among health care professionals. This impacts directly on the ability of lesbian, gay and bisexual people to access health care[32].

Sexual ill health such as STIs or sexual problems, while enormously common, is still shrouded in stigma and embarrassment. People note that it is not like having a cold or flu – it's to do with 'below the waist'. Such issues impact directly on poor emotional and physical health. People with worries around STIs repeatedly say that they feel – *nervous, exposed, vulnerable or scared.* This inhibits them from accessing information, help and treatment. Women will often bypass general practice due to fearing judgemental or negative attitudes by the GP or worrying about confidentiality:
"He knows my family."
"She is my husband's doctor too."
"Ooh I couldn't see my own doctor."

This results in women being prompted to only use a service when symptoms (pain, discomfort during sex, discharge) do not go away and become increasingly intolerable, inexplicable or frightening[33]. Specialist genitourinary medicine (GUM) clinics to which many women can be referred or can self- refer are not always liked either:

"I'm not going down there, it's degrading, they stick your legs in them bloody stirrups."

However, word of mouth about good services has enormous potential to support use:

"I send everyone here because I come here myself."

Consumers views, fears and expectations about GUM services are often quite different to contraceptive services. GUM is seen as *"that sort of place. . . where filthy men go . . ."*[34] as against contraceptive settings which are perceived as nicer, safer and removed from the 'disease' model of health care. Such views need challenging and require knowledge and understanding by all professionals about the role of different sexual health services available in order to improve access and uptake by consumers.

How people access help can be difficult as UK sexual health services are currently fragmented and are split between general practice, community family planning, sexual health and genitourinary clinics and gynaecology services. The pharmacist – an essential member of the primary care team – is an important provider of sexual and reproductive health information. Research shows that when consumers make a decision about who to go to, they make a series of 'trade-offs' – often forgoing privacy in pharmacy settings in favour of easier access to medicines or to avoid examinations[35]. This 'silo' provision of health services is in direct contrast to the needs of women and men who do not come with isolated problems. For instance, a woman requesting emergency contraception has a number of sexual health issues that need support:

- an immediate need to address the consequences of unprotected sex
- a need to provide information, support and advice around STI
- support around the use of contraception – this may address issues around current use or non-use
- careful exploration around sexual activity – consensual, non-consensual or potential abuse?

As such, professionals working in services need to develop a holistic approach, become more 'person-centred' and understand that sex and its pleasures and consequences involves more than the 'waist down, but hearts and minds too'[36].

IMPROVING SEXUAL HEALTH SERVICE PROVISION

Once the complexities relating to sexual health work are recognised, a number of strategies can be introduced to support the way in which sexual health services are delivered:

Service provision

- Provide accessible, flexible services that really address the diversity of sexual and reproductive health care needs of *your* practice and community.

- Provide services that are designed, developed and delivered on the basis of needs assessment – *involve* users, potential users *and* past users of services.

- Provide up-to-date information about all the services you actually offer – so people *know* about them – what you offer, who offers what, when services are available, appointment or 'walk in', domiciliary/home visit. Use leaflets, websites, local directories and posters to let people know.

- Provide information about the sexual health services you do *not* provide and give information on how people can access those services (for example, STI testing). Will you refer or only signpost?

- Find out and really know about other sexual health services, so you can talk about them from a position of understanding, this should include local pharmacy.

- Ensure all staff (clinical, medical and non-medical) are appropriately trained, updated and properly resourced – utilise different professional skills, strengths and interests to the best advantage.

- Ensure confidentiality in visits, communications and record keeping – be seen to care about this – *display a confidentiality poster*.

- Practice an ethos of equality regarding age, gender, race, sexual orientation and disability.

- Know that your service policies, practices and attitudes are non-judgemental, friendly and supportive.

- Provide if possible a choice of female or male doctor, offer advocacy workers and interpreters where needed.

- Ensure that your premises are welcoming and pleasant and accessible for all abilities.

- Provide sufficient *time* – especially for any first visit (this can be split time between doctor and nurse).

Information, support and counselling

- Recognise that issues to do with sex can be embarrassing and may cause anxiety both for consumers *and* professionals.

- Always provide appropriate, accessible, evidence-guided information – recognise the need not to 'limit' or 'censor' information or overwhelm with too much.

- Provide 'back-up' written information to support verbal advice – *use* **fpa** *sexual health leaflets*.

- Always discuss any harm/risk, benefit *and* uncertainty about any contraceptive method, sexual health procedure or treatment – not as a 'tick' for litigious reasons but because it enables shared decision making and improved choices.

- Use suitable, up-to-date language – that enables and informs, understand the meaning of value-laden words such as 'serious', 'small', 'large', 'significant'. Use statistics that can be understood[37].

- Be a catalyst and facilitator not an 'educator' who tends to tell 'what needs to be done'. *Check out* information needs by asking questions.

- Understand that people need 'permission' to ask questions – listen and respond.

- Pay attention to discussed side effects of contraceptive methods or treatments (whether real or perceived), this can say a lot about a person's concerns or need.

- Increase motivation – be prepared to offer solutions to any practical difficulty being experienced, such as using the pill, or practising safer sex.

- Be accessible through telephone support if more information is wanted[38].

People's understanding and needs in sexual health are complex. Primary care professionals have a central and significant role in providing good information and services which in turn play a key part in promoting improved emotional and physical sexual health of the people in the communities that they serve.

Key messages

- Sexual health services in general practice must be based on the needs assessment of users, potential users and past users, and must truly address the diversity of the local community – men as well as women, people of all ages, sexual orientation, ethnic or cultural background, and abilities.

- Primary care professionals need to develop a holistic approach to sexual health services, and to become more 'person-centred'.

- Fears and misconceptions about GUM services should be challenged by primary care professionals in order to improve access and uptake by consumers of the full range of sexual health services.

- Provide clear information about the services on offer using a range of methods including websites, leaflets, posters and local directories. Also, display a confidentiality poster.

- Ensure that all staff are appropriately trained, updated and resourced in order to provide a service that is accessible and non-judgemental, and that is grounded on principles of good practice.

References

1. Department of Health. *The National Strategy for Sexual Health and HIV*. London: Department of Health 2001.

2. Department of Health. *Effective Commissioning of Sexual Health and HIV Services – A Sexual Health and HIV Commissioning Toolkit for Primary Care Trusts and Local Authorities.* London: Department of Health 2003.

3. Department of Health. *Effective Sexual Health Promotion – A Toolkit for Primary Care Trusts and Others Working in the Field for Promoting Good Sexual Health and HIV Prevention.* London: Department of Health 2003.

4. Faculty of Family Planning and Reproductive Health Care (FFPRHC) of the RCOG. *Service Standards for Sexual Health Services.* London: FFPRHC 2003.

5. Medical Foundation for AIDS and Sexual Health. *Recommended Standards for Sexual Health Services.* London: MedFASH, 2005.

6. Johnson A et al. Sexual behaviour in Britain: partnerships, practices and HIV risk behaviours. *The Lancet,* vol 358, no 9296, 2001, pp1835–42.

7. Wellings K et al. Sexual behaviour in Britain: early heterosexual experience. *The Lancet*, vol 358, no 9296, 2001, pp1843–50.

8. Fenton K et al. Sexual behaviour in Britain: reported sexually transmitted infections and prevalent genital Chlamydia trachomatis infection. *The Lancet*, vol 358, no 9296, 2001, pp1851–54.

9. Department of Health. *Shifting the Balance of Power within the NHS – Securing Delivery.* London, Department of Health, 2001.

10. Department of Health. *Shifting the Balance of Power: The Next Steps.* London, Department of Health, 2002.

11. Department of Health. *Choosing Health: Making Healthy Choices Easier.* Cm 6374. London, TSO, 2004.

12. See note 5 above.

13. Royal College of Obstetricians and Gynaecologists (RCOG). *Patient Involvement in Enhancing Service Provision.* London: RCOG 2002.

14. Chambers R, Drinkwater C and Baoth E. *Involving Patients and the Public: How to do it Better.* (2nd edition) Oxford: Radcliffe Medical Press 2003.

15. Harris J et al. User satisfaction: Measurement and Interpretation. *Journal of Family Planning and Reproductive Health Care,* vol 27, no 1, 2001, pp41–45.

16. Herxheimer A and Ziebland S. DIPEx: fresh insights for medical practice. *Journal of Royal Society of Medicine,* vol 96, no 5, 2003, 209–210.

17. Sherman-Jones A. Young People's perceptions of and access to health advice. *Nursing Times,* vol 99, no 30, 2003, pp32–35.

18. Rogstad K. The mystery shoppers – Young people and sexual health clinics. *Positive Nation*, Issue 99, 2004, pp36–39.

19. Brook Advisory Centres and Egg Research and Consultancy. *Someone with a Smile Would be your Best Bet . . . What Young People Want from Sex Advice Services.* London: Brook Advisory Centres 1998.

20. Teenage Pregnancy Unit. *Best Practice Guidance on the Provision of Effective Contraception and Advice Services for Young People.* London: Teenage Pregnancy Unit 2001.

21. Department of Health. *You're Welcome Quality Criteria: Making Health Services Young People Friendly*. London: Department of Health 2005.

22. Burack R. Young teenager's attitudes towards general practitioners and their provision of sexual health care. *British Journal of General Practice* 2000, vol 50, no 456, pp550–554.

23. Seamark C, Blake S. Concerning women: questionnaire survey of consultations, embarrassment, and views on confidentiality in general practice among women in their teens, thirties and fifties. *Journal of Family Planning and Reproductive Health Care 2005,* vol 31, no 1, pp 31–33.

24. McPherson A, Macfarlane A, Allen J. What do young people want from their GP? *British Journal of General Practice,* vol 46, no 411, 1996, p627.

25. Aguma A. Finding the right sexual health services for young men. *Planned Parenthood Challenges* no 2, 1996, pp26–29.

26. Men's Health Forum. *Private Parts, Public Policy. Improving Men's Sexual Health – a Report by the Men's Health Forum.* 2003.

27. Pearson S. Promoting sexual health services to young men: Findings from focus group discussions. *Journal of Family Planning and Reproductive Health Care*, vol 29, no 4, 2003, pp194–98.

28. Bashall R. Disabled women's access to health information – a human rights issue. *Women's Health Newsletter*, no 58, 2003, pp14–15.

29. Qureshi B. Transcultural aspects of family planning and reproductive healthcare. *Journal of Family Planning and Reproductive Health Care,* vol 27, no 1, 2001, pp3–5.

30. Peate I. Sexuality and sexual health promotion for the older person. *British Journal of Nursing,* vol 13, no 4, 2004, pp188–93.

31. See note 16 above.

32. Douglas Scott S, Pringle A and Lumsdaine C. *Sexual Exclusion – Homophobia and Health Inequalities: A Review.* London: UK Gay Men's Health Network 2004.

33. Dixon-Woods M et al. Choosing and using services for sexual health: a qualitative study of women's views. *Sexually Transmitted Infections,* vol 77, no 5, 2001, pp335–39.

34. Scoular A, Duncan B and Hart G. 'That sort of place . . . where filthy men go . . .'. A qualitative study of women's perceptions of genitourinary medicine services. *Sexually Transmitted Infections*, vol 77, no 5, 2001, pp340–43.

35. Ambler S. General practitioners and community pharmacists: times they are a-changing. *British Journal of General Practice*, vol 53, no 493, 2003, pp594–95.

36. Belfield T. Food for thought . . . it's now time to talk. *Journal of Family Planning and Reproductive Health Care*, vol 28, no 2, 2002, p57.

37. Calman K and Royston G. Risk language and dialects. *British Medical Journal,* vol 315, no 7113, 1997, pp939–42.

38. Belfield T. Adapted from: The contraceptive decision: information and counselling (Chap 13) in *Contraception and Office Gynecology. Choices in Reproductive Healthcare.* Editors Kubba A, Sanfilippo J and Hampton N. London: W B Saunders 1999.

Further information

fpa leaflets on STIs

- Your sexual health – where to go for help and advice
- Chlamydia
- Genital herpes
- Genital warts
- Gonorrhoea
- HIV
- Pubic lice and scabies
- Syphilis
- Trichomonas vaginalis
- Vaginal infections (thrush and BV)

fpa leaflets on contraception

- Abortion Your questions answered

Your guide to . . .

- After you've had your baby
- Bodyworks
- The combined pill
- Contraception
- The contraceptive implant
- Contraceptive injections
- The contraceptive patch
- Diaphragms and caps
- Emergency contraception
- Family planning services
- The IUD
- The IUS
- Male and female condoms
- Male and female sterilisation
- Natural family planning
- The progestogen-only pill

Available from **fpa**
Tel: 0845 122 8600
Fax: 0845 123 2349
Email: fpadirect@fpa.org.uk
www.fpa.org.uk

Chapter 11

EVALUATING SEXUAL HEALTH SERVICE PROVISION IN GENERAL PRACTICE

Kaye Wellings

INTRODUCTION

Unplanned pregnancy, sexually transmissible infections (STIs) and HIV, and sexual dysfunction have important consequences for health status, as this volume has repeatedly highlighted. In the general practice setting it is important to know how services might best be provided to reduce adverse outcomes of sexual activity, and to enhance sexual wellbeing. Evaluation research helps to assess the extent to which services are successful in achieving these aims and how best they might be provided. In addition, it helps to assess whether there are any unintended, and possibly undesirable, outcomes.

We need to know which sexual health interventions are effective so that individual practitioners, health authorities and policy makers can decide whether to continue them in their present form or, in the case of novel interventions or pilot projects, whether to adopt them more widely. In the context of limited resources for health-related interventions, evaluation is necessary to establish which ways of working are most cost-effective[1]. Thus an evaluation may be carried out in order to monitor and assess the effect of the existing configuration and provision of services. Or it may be carried out to monitor a new initiative and to assess the extent to which it meets its goals. In practice, and certainly ideally, the two should merge seamlessly so that, should current practice be evaluated and found wanting, an intervention could be designed to meet the unmet need.

THE EVALUATION PROCESS: STAGES OF RESEARCH

For this reason, it is useful to think of evaluation in a number of stages. Evaluation research typically begins with a **developmental component**, in which the potential for service improvement or innovation in clinical practice is explored, along with (wherever possible) identification of factors that might facilitate or obstruct delivery. This is followed by a **formative evaluation**, conducted in order to maximise the appropriateness, acceptability and consistency of an intervention. A **process evaluation** is undertaken during the course of the service delivery or intervention to assess what was done and how, and finally, an **outcome evaluation** is carried out to examine effects, effectiveness and efficacy. If effectiveness is demonstrated and the service continues, routine monitoring and audit subsequently ensure quality of service delivery and continued efficacy.

Ideally, the evaluation process should be continuous. Development of the research and evaluation process is optimally seen, not as linear, but circular, that is, data from the outcome stage of evaluation will feed back into further developments in service delivery, closing the 'loop'.

Developmental research

Research designed to develop service improvement or innovation is generally aimed at identifying and assessing needs which are not being adequately served in general practice. Such research does not need to be, and rarely is, dedicated research carried out specifically to answer these questions. More often, existing research is used opportunistically to reveal service needs.

These needs may be those of health professionals. For example, research has identified practice nurses as having an important role in the provision of sexual health services in general practice, but also that they need more training in the area to fulfil their potential[2].

More often, development research focuses on the needs of patients. In so doing, it may uncover an area of sexual health need which is insufficiently well met in general practice. Studies have, for example, identified barriers in the management of problems of sexual dysfunction expressed by both patients[3,4] and practitioners[5,6]. Despite its prevalence in the population, sexual dysfunction frequently goes undetected in general practice, perhaps because in thinking about sexual health needs the emphasis has tended to be on preventing adverse outcomes of sexual activity – unplanned pregnancy and infection[7] – and less on enabling individuals to achieve fulfilling sexual relationships.

Research has also shown prevention to be another area of neglect in sexual health service provision in general practice. Primary care has the potential to play an important role in promoting sexual health, but studies have shown that many GPs find it difficult to raise sexual health matters in a general consultation and rarely provide advice on safer sex or counselling regarding STIs[8,9,10].

Development research can also assist in targeting at-risk patients. One study, for example,[11] showed that teenage women who attended for termination of pregnancy were more likely to have consulted for emergency contraception or urinary tract symptoms, to have begun using contraception at an early age, to have presented with side effects or dissatisfaction with contraception, to be lapsed users of contraception and to have had a previous pregnancy. These markers of risk can help primary care professionals to identify patients who might be at higher risk of unintended pregnancy, and to take opportunistic preventive action before the risk occurs.

Alternatively, development research might be aimed at determining whether a particular sexual health service is needed at all in general practice, and whether it might not be better met in another service. A considerable body of literature has been amassed examining the balance of contraception in general practice and community based family planning clinics, generally concluding that the two types of service complement, rather than duplicate, one another[12,13].

A common starting point in a systematic evaluation of service delivery is an investigation into the needs of patients. Research into users' views of services is essential in tailoring the service to their needs. An important outcome therefore is patient satisfaction. It is possible[14] and often necessary, in assessing satisfaction with a specific practice, for the research to take place in the same setting as the population served by it. There are, however, good reasons why this should not be the only research strategy.

A sample of patients drawn from the register of a particular general practice being evaluated will consist of patients who continue to frequent that practice and so are more likely to be satisfied customers. If the aim is to explore why people choose particular services, general practice settings are not suitable, since by virtue of being there the patients have chosen this setting in preference to other specialist services for sexual health. As a result, the practice-based sample may under-represent dissatisfied customers and will certainly exclude non-users. Moreover, the fact that patients are on their GPs' premises is likely to inhibit frank appraisal, and they may be fearful of any unfavourable comments they may make, impacting on their own treatment by the practitioner.

Ideally, research needs to be based on a sample representing a broad cross section of young people. Educational settings have been used to good effect in this respect (though they may under-represent the sample of young people who are poor attenders, a group also known to be at risk in terms of sexual health). Investigations which have used the school setting have revealed strong opinions about the type of GP young people would like to consult and the style of surgery they would prefer to attend[15]. Factors influencing presentation for sexual health-related matters have been shown to include concerns about sensitive issues such as confidentiality[16], embarrassment and discomfort[17], unfriendly staff, and delays in getting an appointment[18,19]. A strong conclusion of many of these studies has been that work is needed to improve teenagers' awareness of, and access to, services. In addition, a consideration of factors that might facilitate or obstruct their delivery will assist in providing improved contraceptive services to teenagers.

Simulated clients or 'mystery shoppers', an evaluation strategy more commonly used in market research, is another possible approach to evaluating the limitations of health services and to identify areas that could be addressed to improve patient satisfaction[20]. Another solution to identifying the 'non-user' in general practice is to examine the views of those seeking their sexual health services elsewhere[21]. An important policy question in this context is how user-satisfaction in general practice compares with that in other service settings, for example, family planning, sexual health and genitourinary medicine (GUM). Research which aims to answer this question must necessarily seek a sample using the alternative services. Triggered by concern that GPs' services may be underused for HIV testing, for example, Madge et al (1999)[22] asked attenders at a same-day testing clinic to explain their preference for that service setting. It emerged that the main barriers to using primary care were concerns over the recording of sensitive information in notes, future life insurance and confidentiality, and the fact that GPs rarely discussed HIV testing.

Formative evaluation
Formative research, as stated above, is conducted in order to maximise the appropriateness, acceptability and consistency of an intervention, often prior to an evaluation of its effectiveness. An important goal of the formative phase of evaluation is to identify possible barriers to implementation and to anticipate unforeseen outcomes. One component of formative research is the pre-testing of an intervention to gauge the potential for mishap before full and final application. In practice, where large and complex interventions are introduced into general practice and other service settings, this may take the form of evaluation of a pilot scheme introduced before rolling out the programme more widely. This affords the opportunity to fine tune in readiness for wider uptake.

The recent introduction of opportunistic screening for Chlamydia trachomatis in the UK, and its evaluation in general practice, provides an illustration. As discussed in Chapter 9, in 1999, the UK Department of Health introduced a pilot opportunistic chlamydia screening programme. The aim was to assess its feasibility in reducing the prevalence of, and morbidity associated with, genital chlamydial infection in the UK. Sexually active women attending general practices and other health care settings, such as family planning clinics, antenatal clinics and GUM services, were offered the opportunity to be screened for chlamydia regardless of the purpose of their visit.

In the context of general practice, information was needed about the justification for using this setting; who, when, and how to test; what the costs and benefits were likely to be; and what factors might enhance or impede the process. In such cases, multi-faceted, multi-method evaluation research is needed to answer all the important questions comprehensively. To answer the question relating to justification, one study[23], for example, used screening data from a pilot in different settings – general practice, family planning, GUM, adolescent sexual health, abortion clinics and women's services in hospitals. The study concluded that the relatively high prevalence rate, of approximately 9 per cent in general practice, justified opportunistic screening in general practice as an appropriate method of reaching individuals with infection who do not normally present at specialist clinics.

A multi-faceted research project, the Chlamydia Screening Studies (ClaSS)[24], focused on the feasibility of the scheme in general practice, using several interlinked studies. Results showed, that although mailing of specimens for chlamydia testing appeared to be feasible, it was difficult to achieve high response rates with postal screening. It also revealed a high prevalence of asymptomatic infection in men, prompting the recommendation that efforts to screen men for chlamydia should be strengthened. A further study[25] aimed at assessing feasibility focused on the acceptability of the scheme amongst health professionals in general practice. In-depth interviews with staff revealed that receptionists, whose involvement was central to the opportunistic screening in general practice, nevertheless reported being drawn into discussions for which they felt ill-equipped and unsuitably located. It was this aspect of the model that raised most concerns.

Another research team[26] examined possible barriers to implementation, against a backcloth of wide variation in diagnostic testing by general practice. Using focus group discussions with health professionals, barriers to opportunistic chlamydia testing in general practice were identified as lack of knowledge of the diagnostic procedures and of the benefits of testing; lack of time; and lack of guidance. More crucially, perhaps, for the success of the scheme, these researchers found that none of the practices were happy to discuss chlamydia in a consultation unrelated to sexual health[27]. This prompted them to issue a warning that efforts to increase chlamydia screening in the general practice setting should be accompanied by clear guidance and education, and support from GUM clinics in the provision of appropriate contact tracing and follow-up.

From these multi-faceted enquiries emerges a comprehensive picture of how screening for Chlamydia trachomatis might best be organised and delivered. This includes an understanding of the barriers to effective implementation in general practice. Such research, aimed at formative evaluation, prevents more costly and harmful mistakes being made at a later date and protects the public health and purse from wider investment in projects that are unlikely to be optimally effective.

Process evaluation

Process evaluation focuses on how an intervention will be delivered, answering the question 'What is, or what has happened in the intervention?' This is an important question. If attention was focused simply on the success of the intervention in terms of outcomes, it would not be possible to tell why it worked, or what part of it worked. Thus process evaluation often focuses on input and throughput, on what resources were spent and how, and on how many and which patients benefited or were exposed to the intervention. An important question in this context is which patients were *not* reached, since they may be those on whom the impact of the intervention/service would have been greatest and who might have benefited most.

While outcome evaluation focuses on the extent to which the intended goals of a particular service have been met, process evaluation has valuable potential in helping to uncover unintended consequences of intervention.

Specific issues to be addressed in process evaluation include:

- How well were resources allocated and disseminated?
- Were there any adverse side-effects of the intervention?
- Was there harmony between the needs and expectations of patients and professionals?
- Were there any professional dynamics that interfered with the ways in which the service could optimally be delivered?
- Were there alliances between different interventions or environmental factors which enhanced outcomes?

Process evaluation is often narrowly conceived in terms of measuring 'dose' or exposure, and in this sense more closely resembles audit. Because process evaluation focuses on input and throughput, routine audit data will certainly be used. But research with this aim also needs to focus on the social processes at work in delivery of the service or intervention, on the medical encounter between patients and practitioners, and on the interaction between practitioners themselves.

Outcome evaluation

Process evaluation can answer important questions about the factors influencing the provision and delivery of an intervention, and why something does or does not happen effectively. But ultimately the process has to be linked with the endpoints or outcomes, and the question asked 'Did it work?'

To a large extent, this question is likely to be dependent on the outcomes we choose to measure. The choice of outcome measures is determined by the aims and objectives of interventions. As we have seen, sexual health interventions in general practice may take one of many forms. The intervention may seek to change behaviours; to change prescribing patterns; to improve detection or diagnosis of STI, sexual dysfunction, or unplanned pregnancy; or to change the configuration or organisation of service provision. It may be directed towards patients, with the aim of better meeting their needs, or it may be directed towards health care professionals, with the aim of improving practice. It may involve face-to-face communication; a computerised decision-making tool for patients; or it may involve a therapeutic intervention – the introduction of a new treatment, or a different method of prescribing an existing treatment.

All such initiatives have the broader aim of improving sexual health status, so however diverse their more immediate objectives, ultimately we would expect to see an improvement in sexual wellbeing and/or a reduction in the adverse outcomes of sexual behaviour. However, to measure only those outcomes that match the broader aims of the intervention may be to risk condemning it to apparent failure. This may be because the relationship between what is being done in the intervention and the endpoint is too indirect, or because it needs to be combined with other things for maximum effect. We may, for example, assume that there will be a relationship between provision of contraception in general practice and a reduction in the prevalence of unplanned pregnancy in the practice population. Yet there are many other influences on unplanned pregnancy rates besides what goes on in general practice, and it may not be possible to attribute any subsequent reduction in rates solely to the intervention in general practice.

As a result, outcome measures which determine the ultimate success or failure of an intervention – such as incidence of STI or unplanned pregnancy – may well feature among those measured in general practice. But we also need to include outcomes which correspond to more immediate objectives. In practice, a variety of endpoints is needed, some near to the intervention, some intermediate and others more long term, the assumption being that all these outcomes are related causally to the final outcome.

The selection of outcome measures should therefore be based on a clear hypothesis. For example, to evaluate a general practice intervention which aimed to increase uptake of condoms among those at risk of STIs, valid short term measures might include professional attitudes towards and patients' knowledge of any change in provision. Intermediate indicators might include uptake of condom provision and the long-term outcome would be a reduction in the incidence of infections. Outcomes relating to proximate points along the causal pathway – modification of attitudes or improvement of skills of health professionals, patient satisfaction and quality of care – are more feasible but less attractive in terms of 'proof' of effectiveness; while long term endpoints are more attractive in terms of scientific rigour, but success in achieving them is less assured.

Outcomes should also be those in which the rate of change is likely to be detectable. If the indicator of outcome has a very low prevalence in the population being studied, for example injecting drug use, then statistical power may be insufficient to prove that an intervention is effective. This could have lasting policy implications if the consequence was that no change could be detected. Biological markers can be used to determine any change in rate of STI as a result of an intervention. But some biological measures are not suitable for measuring the outcome of interventions in general practice. The incidence of those STIs which can be treated or which resolve spontaneously, such as Chlamydia trachomatis, Neisseria gonorrhoea and Treponema pallidum (syphilis), can be reduced by improving diagnosis and treatment services without any behavioural change. However, others such as HSV-2, HIV, and HPV are caused by viruses and are incurable so that the organism remains in the body. Consequently, population rates will not be altered by diagnosis and treatment of infected individuals.

A vital question for evaluation is how large the effect has to be in order to make the case for the intervention having worked. Assumptions about the likely extent of change from baseline will determine sample size calculations for the study. Gains made in general practice may be modest because of the size of the target population. Effects will be smaller where the target group is a large

THE HANDBOOK OF SEXUAL HEALTH IN PRIMARY CARE

and heterogeneous mass and it may be at the level of subgroup activity that achievements become observable, hence the importance of disaggregating data by groups of interest.

Changes brought about as a result of an intervention may also be small because the wrong level of objective, and therefore endpoint, has been chosen. In some instances, for example, where the endpoints are too narrowly conceived in terms of biological outcomes, or where measures of morbidity and mortality are used as outcomes in interventions aimed at the general population, the sample may need to be unfeasibly large, and the scale of effect may still be too small to interpret. However, although difficult to interpret, and even if unpromising when looked at from an individual perspective, small effects can be important in public health terms.

Supposing we take a practice, of say 10,000 patients. Fewer than 500 will be in the target group of women aged 13–17. Given a nationwide prevalence of under 18 conceptions of 40 per 1,000 women per year, we could expect 20 women in that practice under the age of 18 to become pregnant. A very large study would be needed to detect statistically significant changes in the conception rate.

Where prevalence of outcome is low, behavioural measures play an important role in assessing the efficacy of an intervention. Even where biological measures are feasible, behavioural measures such as health seeking practices, risk behaviour and risk reduction practice such as condom or contraceptive use can help assess the impact of an intervention. Use of self-reported data has drawbacks in terms of accuracy and validity. However, these can be minimised and reliable responses obtained if a non-judgmental approach is used, if reassurances are given about anonymity, confidentiality and the use to which the data will be put, and if the credentials of the researcher are given.

Combining behavioural and clinical measures also offers potential for triangulation, helping to verify inferences drawn from self-reported data, despite methodological and scientific difficulties. One solution to the problem of bias in the collecting process has been to attempt to triangulate results, or to cross-validate against other data sources which might provide more objective measures of behavioural change. A good deal of information is available in this respect at relatively low cost and might include condom sales figures, screening uptake, helpline statistics, and morbidity and mortality data.

Another major challenge in assessing efficacy is that of attributing outcome to intervention: that is, ensuring that the apparent observed effects are truly the outcome of the general practice intervention or service and not the result of other influences, such as local preventive interventions. The discrete contribution of the general practice intervention may be difficult to assess. Influences on our behaviour are multiple and the biggest changes in behaviour, and hence health status, are likely to come about through forces other than clinical interventions.

Randomised controlled trials

The most rigorous way of attributing outcome to intervention is to use an experimental approach such as a randomised controlled trial or RCT, in which populations or groups of people are randomly allocated either to a group exposed to the intervention, or to a control group not exposed to the intervention, and the two groups compared over time. RCTs are widely accepted as the most reliable method of determining effectiveness – some would argue the only legitimate way of carrying out evaluation. The appeal of the experimental approach depends on being able to ensure that observed differences in outcomes between treatment and control group are not the result of factors other than those associated with the intervention under investigation. This is the best way of being sure that any effects are not the result of forces other than those associated with the intervention.

Yet despite being the most rigorous method of evaluation, RCTs are not applicable in every case. Such evaluations are relatively rare in general practice for a number of reasons. It is often not possible to allocate patients randomly to exposure and control groups, and there may be practical, ethical and in some cases economic reasons for not doing so. There may also be problems in generalising, since effects may be dependent on specific local circumstances that may not be transferable to other practices, or the practice under assessment at some time in the future.

The evidence from RCTs of the effectiveness of interventions aimed at improving sexual health has been disappointing. One study revealed that out of nearly 300 reports of sexual health interventions only three reliably showed an increase in condom use[28]. It is not surprising then that experimental approaches to evaluating sexual health services in general practice have also failed to show significant effects in the relevant outcomes. One of the few cluster randomised trials of condom promotion[29] that have been carried out in general practice looked at whether women being given condoms and STI advice when they attended for smear tests affected subsequent condom use. Although more women in the intervention than control practices reported receiving advice on avoiding STIs and being given condoms, no difference was found in subsequent condom use, even in those reporting more than two sexual partners in the previous year. The authors concluded that, to provide evidence of effectiveness, future interventions may need to focus on higher risk groups.

With considerable NHS investment going into sexual health promotion, there remains an urgent need for reliable evidence of the effectiveness of specific sexual health interventions in general practice. Other design options include:

- before and after designs, following up a cohort of patients or practitioners over time
- area comparisons (comparing practices with and without interventions)
- case control studies (comparing populations exposed with those not so exposed).

All of these are less rigorous than randomised controlled trials. Cost data are also increasingly collected as outcomes, because health technologies have to demonstrate cost effectiveness as well as efficacy to be recommended for adoption by the NHS.

Key messages

- In general practice, evaluation research can help to assess how services might best be provided to reduce adverse outcomes of sexual activity and enhance sexual wellbeing.
- Evaluation should be a continuous process, with data from the outcome stage of evaluation feeding back into further developments in service delivery.
- Research into users' views of services is essential in tailoring the service to their needs.
- While outcome evaluation focuses on the extent to which the intended goals of a service have been met, process evaluation focuses on how they have been met, and is valuable in helping to uncover unintended consequences of an intervention.
- Randomised control studies are widely accepted as the most reliable method of determining effectiveness.

References

1. Ernst E. How much of general practice is based on evidence? *British Journal of General Practice*, vol 54, no 501, 2004, p316.

2. Stokes T and Mears J. Sexual health and the practice nurse: a survey of reported practice and attitudes. *British Journal of Family Planning*, vol 26, no 2, 2002, pp89–92.

3. Gott M and Hinchliff S. Barriers to seeking treatment for sexual problems in primary care: a qualitative study with older people. *Family Practice,* vol 20, no 6, 2003, pp690–95.

4. Kitai E et al. Erectile dysfunction – the effect of sending a questionnaire to patients on consultations with their family doctor. *Family Practice,* vol 19, no 3, 2002, pp247–250.

5. Humphery S and Nazareth I. (2001) GPs' views on their management of sexual dysfunction. *Family Practice,* vol 18, no 5, 2001, pp516–18.

6. Read S, King M and Watson J. (1997) Sexual dysfunction in primary medical care: prevalence, characteristics and detection by the general practitioner. *Journal of Public Health Medicine,* vol 19, no 4, 1997, pp387–91.

7. Cowan F M and Plummer M. Biological, behavioural and psychological outcome measures. Chap 8 in Stephenson J M, Imrie J and Bonell C (ed). *Effective Sexual Health Interventions*. Oxford: Oxford University Press, 2003.

8. Ross J D and Champion J. How are men with urethral discharge managed in general practice? *International Journal of STD and AIDS,* vol 9, 1998, vol 4, pp192–95.

9. Verhoeven V et al. Discussing STIs: doctors are from Mars, patients from Venus. *Family Practice,* vol 20, no 1, 2003, pp11–15.

10. Hinchliff S, Gott M and Galena E. GPs' perceptions of the gender-related barriers to discussing sexual health in consultations – a qualitative study. *European Journal of General Practice*, vol 10, no 2, 2004, pp56–60.

11. Churchill D et al. Teenagers at risk of unintended pregnancy: identification of practical risk markers for use in general practice from a retrospective analysis of case records in the United Kingdom. *International Journal of Adolescent Medicine and Health*, vol 14, no 2, 2002, pp153–60.

12. Singleton C D and Reuter S. (1999) Dual provision or duplication? A survey of family planning provision. *British Journal of Family Planning*, vol 25, no 2, 1999, pp41–44.

13. Bardsley M et al. Estimating the balance of general practice versus family planning clinic coverage of contraceptive services in London. *British Journal of Family Planning,* vol 26, no 1, 2000, pp 21–25.

14. Milne A and Chesson R. (2000) Health services can be cool: partnership with adolescents in primary care. *Family Practice,* vol 17, no 4, 2000, pp305–8.

15. Jones R et al. How can adolescents' needs and concerns best be met? *British Journal of General Practice,* vol 47, no 423, 1997, pp631–34.

16. Doherty L. New approaches to sexual health services in a rural health board area. *International Journal of STD and AIDS,* vol 11, no 9, 2000, pp594–98.

17. Harden A and Ogden J. Sixteen to nineteen year olds' use of, and beliefs about, contraceptive services. *British Journal of Family Planning*, vol 24, no 4, 1999, pp141–44.

18. Donovan C et al. Teenagers' views on the general practice consultation and provision of contraception. *British Journal of General Practice,* vol 47, 1997, no 424, pp715–18.

19. Burack R. Young teenagers' attitudes towards general practitioners and their provision of health care. *British Journal of General Practice*, vol 50, no 456, 2000, pp550–54.

20. Moriarty H, McLeod D and Dowell A. (2003) Mystery shopping in health service evaluation. *British Journal of General Practice*, vol 53, no 497, 2003, pp942–46.

21. Dixon-Woods M et al. Choosing and using services for sexual health: a qualitative study of women's views. *Sexually Transmitted Infections,* vol 77, no 5, 2001, pp335–39.

22. Madge S et al. (1999) Do people attending a same day testing clinic discuss their need for a HIV test with their GP? *British Journal of General Practice,* vol 49, no 447, 1999, pp813–15.

23. Pimenta J M et al. Opportunistic screening for genital chlamydial infection. II: prevalence among healthcare attenders, outcome, and evaluation of positive cases. *Sexually Transmitted Infections*, vol 79, no 1, 2003, pp22–7.

24. Low N et al. The chlamydia screening studies: rationale and design. *Sexually Transmitted Infections,* vol 80, no 5, 2004, pp342–48.

25. Perkins E, Carlisle C and Jackson N. Opportunistic screening for Chlamydia in general practice: the experience of health professionals. *Health and Social Care in the Community,* vol 11, no 4, 2003, pp314–20.

26. McNulty et al. Diagnosis of genital chlamydia in primary care: an explanation of reasons for variation in chlamydia testing. *Sexually Transmitted Infections*, vol 80, no 3, 2004, pp207–11.

27. McNulty et al. Barriers to opportunistic chlamydia testing in primary care. *British Journal of General Practice,* vol 54, no 504, 2004, pp508–14.

28. Oakley A et al. Sexual health interventions for young people: a methodological review. *BMJ,* vol 310, no 6973, 1995, pp158–162.

29. Oakeshott P et al. Condom promotion in women attending inner city general practices for cervical smears: a randomized controlled trial. *Family Practice*, vol 17, no 1, 2000, pp56–59.

About the authors and editors

Toni Belfield BSc (Hons), FRSH, Hon Fellow FFPRHC, is Director of Information at **fpa**. She is also a member of the RCOG Consumers' Forum and the RCOG Patient Information Group, as well as providing consumer representation for the Cochrane Fertility Regulation Group and other UK and European organisations working in contraception and sexual health.

Yvonne Carter OBE, MD, FRCGP, FMedSci, is Dean of Warwick Medical School, the University of Warwick. She is also Professor of General Practice and Primary Care, a practising general practitioner in Coventry, and a Non-Executive Director at the University Hospitals Coventry and Warwickshire NHS Trust.

Caroline Davey BA (Hons), is the Policy Manager at **fpa**, responsible for the organisation's policy and parliamentary work. She formerly worked in social research and policy in both the private and voluntary sectors.

Muir Gray CBE, DSc, MD, FRCP, FRCPGlas, is Director of Clinical Knowledge, Process and Safety for Connecting for Health and Programmes Director of the UK National Screening Committee.

Kate Guthrie FRCOG, MFFP, is Clinical Director/Consultant in Sexual and Reproductive Health of the Sexual and Reproductive Health Care Partnership for Hull and East Yorkshire. Abortion care is one of her lead service activities. She chaired the Faculty of Family Planning special skills working party to develop a training programme in abortion care, and has recently been appointed to the Independent Advisory Group on Sexual Health as a provider of abortion services.

Philip Hannaford MD, MRCGP, MFFP, DCH, DRCOG, is NHS Grampian Professor of Primary Care. In his current post, his main responsibility is to facilitate research within primary care. Main research interests include women's health issues, the health effects of oral contraception and hormone replacement therapy, primary care epidemiology, and how research and data inform clinical practice.

Tom Heyes MA, MB, BChir, DRCOG, FRCGP, is Clinical Director of General Practice development in Leeds West PCT. Qualifying as a general practitioner in 1984, he has worked for 20 years in partnerships and single handed practice. He was given a grant by Trent NHSE to research preconception care and carried out a three-year project conducting a randomised controlled trial and a survey of primary care workers.

Jennifer Hopwood, FFFP, DipVen, is a specialist working in sexual health services including contraception. She has been closely involved with the cervical screening programme, including taking smears, as a cervical cytologist and as a colposcopist. She has spent almost 20 years in collaborative research and in the development of chlamydia detection, leading to the implementation of a community-wide screening programme.

Rita Ireson BA, PGDip, MSc, is Co-manager of the Sexual Health Promotion Service at the Heart of Birmingham Teaching Primary Care Trust. She is a sexual health promotion specialist with particular focus on the primary care setting. She has wide experience as a trainer and lecturer in sexual health, and is currently an associate lecturer at Warwick University.

Helen Macaulay RN, is a sexual health outreach worker based in primary care. She is currently working on a project which aims to support the delivery of sexual health services in primary care. This involves training general practitioners and practice nurses, developing sexual health guidelines and providing open access clinics for young people.

Philippa Matthews FRCGP, is a general practitioner in Lee Bank Group Practice, Birmingham. She leads the SHOW project, which provides integrated sexual health care to those at highest risk. She developed the Sexual Health in Primary Care postgraduate award at the University of Warwick, commissioned by the West Midlands Deanery.

Shelley Mehigan SRN, OHNC, Extended Nurse Prescriber is a clinical nurse specialist in family planning, working in sexual health clinics in East Berkshire, and in general practice in Maidenhead. She has worked in general practice for 20 years, specialising in family planning for 18 years. She contributed to the Crown Review of Prescribing.

Catti Moss FRCGP, is a general practitioner in rural Northamptonshire, and a part-time clinical lecturer at Warwick Medical School, University of Warwick. She is a general practitioner trainer and appraiser. She is also Medical Vice Chair of the RCGP Patients' Partnership Group.

Catriona Sutherland RN, Extended and Supplementary Prescriber, is a clinical nurse specialist in women's reproductive and sexual health. She works in general practice in South London, and in a community sexual health clinic in Southwark.

Gill Wakley MD, MFFP, MIPM, is a visiting professor in primary care development at Staffordshire University. She also works as a freelance general practitioner, writer and lecturer. Her MD thesis was on providing better sexual health care in primary care.

Kaye Wellings BA, MSC, FRCOG, FFPH, is Professor of Sexual and Reproductive Health at the London School of Hygiene and Tropical Medicine. She has been involved in sexual health research for over 20 years and was a founder of, and Principal Investigator on, the National Surveys of Sexual Attitudes and Lifestyles (Natsal 1990 and 2000). She has been extensively involved in the evaluation of sexual health interventions, including the Government's Teenage Pregnancy Strategy.

Anne Weyman OBE, BSc (Soc), FCA, Doctor of Laws (honorary), is Chief Executive of **fpa**. She is the Founder and Honorary President of the Sex Education Forum, the Vice Chair of the Independent Advisory Group on Sexual Health, and a member of the Independent Advisory Group on Teenage Pregnancy.

Index

Abortion Act (1967)   137, 138

Abortion services

  access to   138-142
    ensuring speedy   139-140, 148
    initial examination   139
    other groups of women   142
    referral   140
    signposting to related services   139
    young women   140-142, 148
  adherence to standards   148-149
  child protection issues   141-142
  confidentiality   139, 148
  contraception   143
  emergency access   139
  Fraser criteria to assess capacity
    to consent   141
  HSA1 certificate   142-143
  key messages   151
  legal aspects
    Isle of Man   152-153
    Northern Ireland   152
    Scotland, England and Wales   137-138
  National Sexual Health Strategies   137, 148
  NHS Plan   137
  organisation   148-149
  patient choice   145, 150
  patient information   143–144,146, 150
  professional practice guidelines   140
  rapid discharge protocol   145
  Recommended Standards for Sexual
    Health Services   138, 148
  referring without delay   142-143
  sexual health screening   143
  statutory grounds for termination
    of pregnancy   138
  summary   150-151
  trained workforce   150
  user/carer representation   150

Abortions   143-145

  chlamydial screening and   237
  complications   145-148
    early post-procedure   147
    failure rates   147
    immediate   146-147
    long-term effects   147-148
  follow-up in primary care   148-149
  maximum waiting times   144-145
  procedures
    according to gestation band   144
    medical regimes   145
    surgical   144, 145
  psychological effects   147, 148
  recommended methods by
    gestation band   144
  and risk of STIs   143
  risk of subsequent abortions   143
  service organisation   149-150

Acquired immune deficiency syndrome
  (AIDS)   190

Acts of Parliament

  Abortion Act 1967   137, 138
  Data Protection Act 1988   200
  Medicines Act 1968   30-31
  Termination of Pregnancy (Medical
    Defences) Act 1995 (Isle of Man)   152-153

AIDS, *see* Acquired Immune
  Deficiency Syndrome

Antenatal screening

  HIV infection   160, 191
  STIs   160
  see also Pregnancy planning

Anti-sperm antibodies, following vasectomy 101

Antibiotics, broad-spectrum

  combined oral contraceptives   85
  contraceptive patch   88

Antimalarials, and ART 206

Antiretroviral therapy (ART) 190, 191
    adherence 204
    interactions 204, 206
    side effects 204

Apomorphine, sublingual (Uprima) 216

ART, see Antiretroviral therapy

Arterial disease, COC and increased risk 78

Arthritis, and sexual dysfunction 224

Association of Psychosexual Nursing 220

Bacterial vaginosis 158, 164

Barrier methods
    advantages
        contraceptive 92
        non-contraceptive 93
    conditions of use
        broadly usable with 93-94
        monitoring during usage 94
        not usable with 93
        use with caution 93
    description 92
    disadvantages 93
    see also Condom

Bisexuality, attitudes to 250

Breast cancer
    abortion and 148
    COC and 78
    progestogen-only implants and 61-62
    screening 234

Breastfeeding
    as contraceptive method 95
    HIV transmission 188

British Pregnancy Advisory Service,
    rapid discharge protocol study 145

Calendar method 94

Call/recall 237

Candida
    diagnostic test 164
    not managed as sexually transmissible 158
    oesophageal 196

Cap, see Barrier methods

Cardiovascular disease, and sexual
    dysfunction 224

Case control studies 269

CD4 count 188-189, 190

Cerazette (progestogen-only pill) 92
    see also Progestogen-only pill

Cervical cancer

contraception
    barrier methods 94
    COC and possible increased risk 78
    screening
        age and timing of 237
        HIV infected patient 205
        inappropriate use for STI screening 238
        incidental finding of STIs 160-161
        less likely in high-risk patients 38
    and sexual dysfunction 224
    smoking and risk 38

Cervical mucus method 94

Child protection
    and abortion services 141-142
    illegal sexual activity 142

Child sexual abuse 53, 218-219

Childbirth, sexual dysfunction after 213-214

Chlamydial infection
(Chlamydia trachomatis)
    clinical consequences 161-162
    conjunctivitis 166-167
    diagnostic tests 163, 165, 166
    incidental finding from urine sample 160-161
    partner notification 170
    prevalence in primary care 36
    prevention of infection 239
    neonatal conjunctivitis 160
    screening
        before IUS insertion 72
        confidentiality of results 241
        deciding who to screen 236, 240
        diagnosis or screening? 240-241
        evaluation of risk 241
        facilitating access 238, 240
        and follow-up 240
        formative evaluation of provision 263-264
        frequency of 240, 241
        funding 241
        measuring population coverage 241
        multidisciplinary and joined-up
           working 241
        national screening programme 161, 240,
        242
        nucleic acid amplification test 239
        screening parameters with respect to 239
        and treatment 239, 240, 242
    sexually transmitted infection 158
    test of cure 171
    vertical transmission to babies 160

Chlamydial Screening Studies (ClaSS) 263

Cialis (tadalafil) 216

Clomiprimine 217

CMV (cytomegalovirus retinitis) 195-196, 198

Colon cancer screening   235

Colostomy, and sexual dysfunction   225

Combined contraceptive patch

   advantages   86

   concomitant use of other drugs   88

   conditions of use

      broadly usable   80-81, 86

      not usable with   78-79, 86

      usable with caution   79-80, 86

   delayed application   87

   description   86

   disadvantages   86

   HIV infected patient   205

   initial assessment before use   86

   main effects   86

   monitoring during usage   87

Combined oral contraceptives (COCs)

   advantages

      contraceptive   77

      non-contraceptive   77

   concomitant use of other drugs

      broad-spectrum antibiotics   85

      liver enzyme-inducing drugs   80, 85

      other drugs   85

   conditions of use

      broadly usable with   80-81

      not usable with   78-79

      usable with caution   79-80

   description   76

   diarrhoea and vomiting   84

   disadvantages   77-78

   follow-up visits   83

   initial assessment before use   82

   main effects   76

   missed pills   83-84

   monitoring during usage   83

   starting   82-83

   surgery   84-85

   travel and risk of DVT   84

Condom

   assessment of use   51

   frenulum tear protected by   213

   prevention of HIV transmission   191, 205

   promotion, randomised trial   268-269

   treatment of premature ejaculation   218

   see also Barrier methods

Confidentiality

   abortion services   139,148

   Data Protection Act 1988   200-201

   importance to consumers   249

Consent, Fraser criteria to assess

   capacity to   141

Contact tracing   168, 169

   see also Partner notification

Contraception

   abortion services and   143

   assessment of use   51

   factors affecting choice   60

      medical conditions   57-58

   history of GP involvement   20

   HIV infected patient   81, 93, 205-206

   improving patient access   31

   information for service providers   58

   lactational amenorrhoea   95

   primary care provision

      benefits of family planning clinic   59

      challenge for   59

      model of good practice   59

   relative effectiveness of methods   60

   sexual dysfunction and   225

   sexually transmitted infections 69, 72, 75-80

   sterilisation   98-101

   use of more than one method   60

   see also Natural family planning/fertility

      awareness; specific methods

Copper-bearing intrauterine devices (IUDs)

   advantages   73

   conditions of use

      broadly usable with   74-75

      not to be used   73-74

      usable with caution   74

   description   73

   disadvantages   73

      emergency contraception   97-98

      HIV infected patient   206

   fitting after abortion   143

   initial assessment before insertion   75-76

   main effects   76

   monitoring during usage   76

   pregnancy occurring with use   76

   removal   76

   timing of insertion   76

Cystic fibrosis screening   234-235

Cytomegalovirus retinitis (CMV)   195-196, 198

Data Protection Act 1988   200-201

   information not to be divulged   201

Depot medroxyprogesterone acetate

   (DMPA, Depo-Provera)   61

   amenorrhoea and weight gain   61

   delayed return to fertility   61, 64

   hypo-estrogenic effects and

      perimenopause   62

   reduced risk of endometrial cancer   61

switching to norethisterone enanthate 64
see also Progestogen-only
    contraceptive injections
Diagnostic tests
    compared with screening   241
    false negative   237
    false positive   237
    sensitivity and specificity
        definitions   236
        method for calculating   237
Diaphragm, see Barrier methods
Dietician, preconceptual care   128
DIPEx (Database of Personal Experience
    of Health and Illness)   248, 250
Disabled people
    abortion services   142
    inadequate service provision   249-250
Diverticular disease, and sexual
    dysfunction   212
DMPA, see Depot medroxyprogesterone acetate
Domestic violence   157, 219, 220
    see also Sexual violence
Drug users
    HIV infection
        increased risk   188
        preventive measures   191
    and sexual dysfunction   226
    and sexual ill-health   38
Dyspareunia, causes of   212-213

Ectopic pregnancy
    as complication of abortion   147
    female sterilisation   99, 100
Ejaculatory difficulties   217-218
    premature ejaculation   217-218
    retarded ejaculation   218
Emergency contraception
    checklist for provision   119
    Concrete Towers Practice guidance   113-118
        access and signposting   113-114
        aims of   113
        hormonal method   114-115
        IUCD   115-117
        missed or late contraception and 117-118
    copper IUD   97-98
    HIV infected patient   206
    hormonal
        advantages   96
        conditions broadly usable with   96
        conditions not to be used with   96
        conditions to be used cautiously with   96
        description   95

disadvantages   96
    initial assessment before use   96-97
    monitoring after usage   97
    sexual health issues associated with   251
Endometrial cancer, COC and reduced risk   77
Endometriosis, intercourse-related pain   212
Enzyme-linked immunosorbent assay
    (ELISA)   165
Epididymal cysts, painful sex and   213
Erectile dysfunction (ED)
    age-related incidence   214
    definition of   214
    examination of man   215
    investigations   215-216
    man's feelings due to   214
    medical conditions associated   214
    responding to complaint of   214
    treatment options
        counselling   216
        hormone replacement   216
        injection therapy   217
        lifestyle changes   216
        medication changes   216
        NHS restrictions   217
        oral therapy   216
        penile prosthesis   217
        surgical   217
        vacuum devices   216-217
Erythromycin   171
Ethnic minorities
    abortion services   142, 144
    sexual health services provision   250
Etonorgestrel (Implanon)   64
Evaluation of sexual health service provision in
    general practice
    developmental research   259, 260-262
        barriers to management of
            sexual dysfunction   260
        drawbacks of GP setting   261
        educational settings   261-262
        family planning provision   261
        other service settings   262
        patients' needs as starting point   261
        prevention as neglected area   260-261
        service improvement   260
        targeting at-risk patients   262
    formative evaluation   260, 262-264
        chlamydial screening as example 263-264
        pilot scheme   262-263
        purpose of   262
    key messages   269
    other research designs
        area comparisons   269
        before and after   269

case control studies 269

outcome evaluation 265-268
attribution to intervention 267-268
behavioural measures affecting 267
choice of outcome 265-266
hypothesis 266
randomised controlled trials 268-269
range of outcomes 266
rate of change of outcome 266
size of effect 266-267
triangulation 267
process evaluation 264-265
audit compared 265
definition of 264
specific issues 264
rationale for 259

Faculty of Family Planning
abortion service standards 149
abortion surgical training programme 150

Familial hypercholesterolaemia 233

fpa
abortion service standards 149
abortion services in Northern Ireland 152
enquiries received by 248
origin 19
patient information on STIs 169, 179
sexual health leaflets 253
young people's views 248-249

Family planning clinics
benefits 59
history of 20

Female genital mutilation 212

Female sterilisation
advantages 99
at time of abortion 143
description 98
disadvantages 99
initial assessment before operation 99-100
post-operative monitoring 100
special precautions 99

Fertility devices for timing ovulation 94

Floaters, associated with CMV retinitis 195, 198

Folic acid supplements 122, 124, 125

Fraser criteria to assess capacity to consent 141

Gardnerella vaginalis infection 158, 164

Gay men,
attitudes to 250
risk of HIV infection 187

Genetic screening, preconceptual 124, 125

Genital herpes
antenatal screening 160
contact tracing not needed 169
diagnosis 162, 164
see also Human papilloma virus

Genital warts 155
clinical diagnosis 162
contact tracing not needed 169

Genitourinary medicine (GUM)
consumers' views about 251
non-attendance and role of GP 172
referral from primary care 171-172
are confidentiality concerns
founded? 172
proposals for future referral model 173-174
quality of care costs due to
informality 172-173
spectrum of risk 37

GMS contract, and sexual health care 20-21

Gonorrhoea (Neisseria gonorrhoea)
condom and reduced transmission 158
conjunctivitis 166
diagnosis 162, 163, 164, 166
bacterial culture 164
partner notification 170
test of cure 171
vertical transmission to babies 158, 160

Haemolytic streptococcus Group B 158, 164

Health Protection Agency, HIV
epidemiological data 188

Health visitor, preconceptual care 128

Hepatitis A, antibody test 165

Hepatitis B
antenatal screening for 160
partner notification 170, 171
post-exposure procedure 184-185
Red Chimneys Practice guidelines
immunisation 183-185
testing 182-183
sexual transmission of 158
testing for 203

Hepatitis C
antibody test 165
partner notification 170, 171
sexual transmission 159

Herpes simplex viruses (HSV I/II)
sexual transmission 158
see also Genital herpes

HIV infection
antenatal screening 160

asymptomatic patients, detection   199-200
caring for patients with
    antiretroviral therapy   204
    cervical screening   205
    contraception   205-206
    drug interactions   205-206
    immunisation   205
    international travel   206
    sexual health advice   205
CD4 count   188-189, 190
communication   192, 199, 201
    implications of positive   202
    readiness to discuss possibility   193, 199
contraceptive use   81, 93, 205
description of virus   188
detection in primary care   191-192, 199-200
diagnosis   162
epidemiology   37, 187-188
immunosuppressed patients
    additional evidence   196-199
    common conditions and
      symptoms   194, 196-198
    HIV testing   199
    learning to recognise   194
    rare conditions more specific to
      HIV   194-196, 196-198
    symptoms   193-194
key messages   206
National Strategy for Sexual Health
    and HIV   246
natural history   188, 189
opportunistic infection   189
P24 antigen test   190, 202
partner notification   170, 171
post-exposure prophylaxis   191
primary or seroconversion   192-193
    HIV antibody test   193
    possible symptoms   193
    risk assessment   193
stigma of   200
STIs and risk of   188
symptomatic patient   192
transmission
    methods of   188
    prevention   191
undiagnosed cases
    primary care   187
    risk to health   187
viral load   189, 190
window period   190
HIV testing
barrier to use of GP services   262
confidentiality   203
consent   203

giving results to patient
    negative test   203
    positive test   203
    immunosuppressed patient   199
    providing patient information   202
HIV testing in primary care
    barriers to testing   200
    medical reports for insurance   200-201
    skills required for   201
    time and resources needed   201-202
    window period   202
HSA1 certificate   142-143
Human papilloma virus (HPV)
    contact tracing   169
    incidental finding on cervical smear   161
    poikilocytosis   161
    sexual transmission   158
    vertical transmission to babies   160
    see also Genital herpes
Hysterectomy, and sexual dysfunction   225

Ileostomy, and sexual dysfunction   225
Immunisation, HIV infected patient   205
Immunosuppressed patients, see under
    HIV infection
Implanon (etonorgestrel)   64
    see also Progestogen-only contraceptives
Infections
    post-abortion   147
    see also Sexually transmitted infections
Insurance reports, see Medical insurance
    reports   201
Irritable bowel syndrome, and sexual
    dysfunction   212
Isle of Man, abortion services   152-153
IUD, see Copper-bearing intrauterine devices
IUS, see Levonorgestrel-releasing intrauterine
    system

Kaposi's sarcoma   195, 196, 197

Lactational amenorrhoea, as
    contraceptive method   95
Learning disabilities, and sexual
    dysfunction   225
Levonorgestrel-releasing intrauterine
    system (IUS)
    advantages
      contraceptive   68
      non-contraceptive   68

conditions of use
  broadly usable with 70-72
  not to be used 69
  theoretical concerns 72
  usable with caution 70
description 68
fitting after abortion 143
initial assessment before insertion 72
liver enzyme-inducing drugs and 72
main effects 68
monitoring during usage 72
STI screening 72
timing of insertion 69, 70
Lignocaine spray, for premature ejaculation 218
Liver enzyme-inducing drugs
  combined oral contraceptive 85
  contraceptive patch 88
  levonorgestrel-releasing IUS and 72
  progestogen-only contraceptive
    implants 66, 67

Male sterilisation
  advantages 100
  description 100
  disadvantages 100-101
  initial assessment before the operation 101
  monitoring after operation 101
  special precautions 101
Mandated 237
Mankind UK 219, 223
Medical insurance reports
  confidentiality 42, 172
  HIV testing and 200-201
  standardised forms 201
Medication
  independent prescribing 31
  patient group directions 31
  Medicines Act 1968 30-31
  and sexual dysfunction 225
  supplementary prescribing 31
  supplying to patients 30
  use of protocols 30-31
Medicines Act 1968 30-31
Men
  inadequate service provision 249
  well man clinic and chlamydia screening 238
Men's Health Forum 249
Menopause, and sexual dysfunction 225
Mental illness, and sexual dysfunction 225
Midwife, preconceptual care 128

Mifepristone 144, 145
Miscarriage, abortion and risk of 148
Mycoplasma genitalum 159

National Birth Control Association (NBCA) 19
  see also **fpa**
National Chlamydia Screening
  Programme 20, 240, 242
  pilots 161
  see also under Chlamydia infection
National Domestic Violence Helpline 223
  see also Domestic violence
National Strategy for HIV and Sexual
  Health 200, 246
  abortion services 149
National Survey of Attitudes and Lifestyles 247
National UK Screening Committee
  criteria 230-231
Natural family planning/fertility awareness
  advantages 94-95
  breastfeeding 95
  description 94
  disadvantages 95
NCSP, see National Chlamydia Screening
  Programme
Needle-stick injuries, post-exposure
  prophylaxis of HIV infection 191
Neisseria gonorrhoea 158
  see also Gonorrhoea
Neonates
  STI-related eye disease 166-167
  vertical transmission of STI 158, 160
NET-EN, see Norethisterone enanthate
Neural tube defects, and folic acid
  supplements 125
NHS Cervical Screening Programme (NHSCSP)
  Call/recall 237
  see also Cervical cancer, screening
NHS Plan
  abortion services 137
  consumers' views important 247
NHS walk-in centre 25
Non-specific urethritis (NSU)
  diagnosis 164
  incidental finding in urine sample 162
  partner notification 170, 171
Nonoxinol-9, and STIs 93
Norethisterone enanthate
  (NET-EN, Noristerat) 61

switching to depot medroxyprogesterone
acetate 64
see also Progestogen-only contraceptive
injections
Norplant (levonorgestrel) 64
see also Progestogen-only contraceptive
implants
Northern Ireland, abortion services 152
Nucleic acid amplification tests 163-164, 239
Nurse prescriber 31
Nursing & Midwifery Council (NMC) 140

Oesophageal candidiasis 196, 197
Older people, and sexuality 250
Opportunistic case finding 237
Opportunistic infections 189
Opportunistic recruitment 237
Oral hairy leukoplakia 195, 197
Ovarian cancer, COC and reduced risk 77
Ovulation, methods of timing 94

P24 antigen test 190, 202
Partner notification
chlamydial screening programmes 240
PID treatment and 169-170, 238
see also Contact tracing
PCP (Pneumocystis carinii
pneumonia) 194-195, 197
Pelvic inflammatory disease (PID)
COC and reduced risk 77
and contraception, copper-bearing
IUDs 75, 76
partner notification 170, 238
Pelvic organs, blood flow and painful sex 213
Penile deformities/infection, and
painful sex 213
Penile prosthesis 217
PEP (post-exposure prophylaxis), for HIV 191
PGDs (patient group directions) 31
Persona (fertility device) 94, 95
Pharmacist
consumer choice for services 251
prescribing 31
Phosphodiesterase type 5 inhibitors 216
PID, *see* Pelvic inflammatory disease
Placenta praevia, sharp curettage and 148
Pneumocystis carinii pneumonia (PCP)
194-195, 197
Poikilocytosis 161

Polymerase chain reaction (PCR) 163
Post-exposure prophylaxis (PEP), for HIV 191
Practice nurse, preconceptual care 128
Preconceptual care, *see* Pregnancy planning
Pregnancy
factors determining outcome 121-122
intercourse during 213
occurring during IUD use 76
unplanned
prior primary care consultation 36
see Abortion services
Pregnancy planning
advice on
dietary issues 124-125
drug dependency treatment 127
environmental hazards 126
medical conditions 125-126
sexual activity 126-127
smoking cessation 127
social support 125
travelling 127
clinical approach 122-129
advice 124-127
audit 128
examination and investigation 124
record-keeping 128
team members 128-129
contacting target audience
local action 129
national policy 130
primary care team level 129
factors determining pregnancy
outcomes 121-122
future research and development 130
history taking
alcohol and drug use 123
anxieties and strengths 123
chronic diseases 124
debriefing/narrative 123
genetic disorders 124
health lifestyle issues 124
immunisation status 124
obstetric history 123
occupational/environmental
hazards 123-124
relationships 123
smoking history 123
key messages 131
links to evidence-based guidelines
and policies 134
useful organisations/websites 134-135
Preterm birth, miscarriage and risk of 148
Professional skill mix
creating effective team 22-23

THE HANDBOOK OF SEXUAL HEALTH IN PRIMARY CARE

history of development of 19-22

future of 28-29, 31-32

general practice with special interest in
sexual health 24

how teams evolve 23

key messages 32

large inner city practice 24

multi-agency approach 28

NHS walk-in centre 25

rural practice 25-26

sexual health service 25

skills and knowledge for primary care 26-27

specialist young people's services 24, 28

urban practice 26

whole practice 27

Progesterone antagonist see Mifepristone

Progestogen-only contraceptive implants
advantages 65

concomitant usage of other drugs 68

description 64-65

disadvantages 65

fitting at time of abortion 143

HIV infected patient 205

main effects 65

and medical conditions
broadly usable with 66-67

initial assessment before insertion 67

not to be used 65

usable with caution 65-66

monitoring during usage 67

timing of insertion 67

Progestogen-only contraceptive
injections 61-64

advantages 61

conditions of use
broadly usable 62-63

not to be used 62

use with caution 62

disadvantages 61-62

initial assessment before injection 63-64

main effects 61

monitoring during usage 64

timing of first injection 64

Progestogen-only pill (POP)
advantages 88

conditions of use
broadly usable with 89-90

not usable with 89

use with caution 89

description 88

diarrhoea and vomiting 92

disadvantages 88-89

follow-up visits 91

initial assessment 90-91

main effects 88

missed pills 92

monitoring during usage 91

Prolapse, and sexual dysfunction 226

Prostaglandin analogue
as abortofacient 144, 145

taken at home 145

Prostate cancer
screening 235

vasectomy and risk of, 101

Prostate enlargement, and sexual
dysfunction 226

Prostitution, and primary care
consultation rate 36

Protocols, for medication 30-31

Psychological effects
of abortion 147, 148

mental illness and sexual
dysfunction 38, 225

Pubic lice 155, 158

diagnosis 162

partner treatment 169

sexual transmission 158

Randomised control trials 268-269

Rape Crisis Federation 219, 223

Recommended Standards and Networks
for Sexual Health Services (DoH,2005) 138

Relate 223

Resolve (Vaginismus Support Group) 223

Risk assessment
how far to take back 53

importance of 35

interpreting 53-54

avoidance of blame on partner 55

future risk and behaviour change 55

moderate to high risk 55

no risk since last test 54-55

patients at no risk 54

patients at very slight risk 54

key messages 56

risk behaviour 35, 37

risk groups 35, 37

unmet need in primary care 36

see also Sexual history-taking

Royal College of Obstetricians and
Gynaecologists (RCOG), abortion service
standards 149

Safer sexual practices 191, 205

St John's wort, *see* Liver enzyme-inducing drugs

Salpingectomy, partial 98

Samaritans 219, 223

Scabies 159, 169

Screening
  abdominal aortic aneurysm 236
  adverse effects of 235
  breast cancer 234
  cervical cancer 237, 238
  colon cancer 235
  concepts
    call-recall 237
    opportunistic case finding 237
    opportunistic recruitment 237
    targeted 237
  criteria for evaluating 230-231
    and course of disease 232
  cystic fibrosis 234-235
  deciding who to screen 236
  for disease 233
    grey zones of disease 234-235
  early enthusiasm in 1960s 228
  elements of a programme 234
  facilitating access 238
  harm versus benefit debate 227-229
  individuals at risk
    with disease 233-234
    and distribution curve 232
    for risk factor 233
  key messages 242
  National UK Screening Committee
    criteria 230-231
  patient, consumer or punter? 235
  prostate cancer 235
  reproducibility of research 228
  risk reduction 236, 242
  screens and sieves 236
  sexual health
    prevention of TFI 238-239
    see also under Chlamydia infection
  Wilson and Jungner criteria 228, 229
  women as traditionally accessible 238
  see also under Chlamydia infection;
    Diagnostic tests

Screens 236

Secondary care specialists,
  preconceptual care 128-129

Selective serotonin reuptake inhibitor
  (SSRI), for premature ejaculation 217

Sensitivity, of test 236

Seroconversion, seroconversion illness 192-193

Sexual Dysfunction Association 223

Sexual dysfunction in primary care
  avoidable errors by GP 209
  chaperone 211
  consultation skills 210-211
  ejaculatory difficulties 217-218
  following childbirth 213-214
  illness or treatment affecting
    sexuality 211-212
    physical effects 211
    psychological affects 211
    treatment, adverse effects of 211-212
  key messages 220
  painful sex in men 213
  painful sex in women 212-213
  presentation 211
  prevalence in general population 209
  referral 220
  sexual violence 218-220
  vaginal fantasies 213
  see also Erectile dysfunction

Sexual health
  National Strategy for Sexual Health
    and HIV 246
  unique role of general practice 246
  user/provider difficulties in addressing 246

Sexual health outreach worker (SHOW)
  project 29-30

Sexual health services
  consumers' views
    confidentiality 249
    difficulty accessing information 248
    DIPEx 248, 250
    disabled 249-250
    embarrassment and stigma 249, 250
    GUM clinic 251
    illness and sexuality 250
    impact on use of 247
    NHS Plan and importance of 247
    older people 250
    poor provision for men 249
    typical queries about 247-248
    visiting pharmacy 251
    visiting their GP 249, 250
    young people's views 248-249
  describing those who use 245
  ethnic and cultural concerns 250
  gender differences in provision 250
  holistic approach important 252, 254
  homosexual and bisexual people 250
  key messages 254
  poor provision for men 249

strategies to improve
    information, support, counselling   253
    service provision   252-253
  unique role of general practice   246

Sexual history-taking
  avoiding inappropriate assumptions   43-44
  benefit for patient   26
  checking understanding   45
  communication
    open/closed questions   42
    patient's distress   42
    patient's agenda   43
    sexual violence   43
  confidentiality   42
  giving information   44
  giving test results   44, 203
  how to carry out   49-55
    asking about sexual practices   50-51
    condom use assessment   51
    contraception assessment   51
    future risk   52
    HIV risk   52
    limitations of symptom questions   49
    miscellaneous questions   52-53
    starting or changing contraception   52
    taking partner history   50
  joining up history   42
  key messages   56
  making judgements   44
  other health issues   38
  see also under specific contraceptive
    methods
    as patient-led   36
  risk behaviours   35, 37
  risk groups   37
  social exclusion issues   38
  spectrum of risk in primary care   37
  strategies for difficulty during   45-48
  those at no risk   39
  why and when to use   39-42
  see also Risk assessment

Sexual lifestyle and behaviour
  directly related factors   247
  wide variability   247

Sexual violence   53, 218-219
  history-taking and   43
  referral to useful organisations   219-220

Sexually transmitted infections (STIs)
  abortion and risk of   143
  asymptomatic
    awareness of possibility of STIs   156
    opportunistic screening   161
    transmission via   161

barrier contraception   93
central role of primary care   155
change in clinical picture in primary care 155
clinical consequences of STIs   161-162
confirming diagnosis
  antibody tests   165
  bacterial culture   164
  chlamydial culture   164
  choice of method and site   166-167
  choice of test   163
  clinical   162
  delay between infection and positive
    test   163
  enzyme-linked immunosorbent assay 165
  genital herpes culture   164
  men with possible genital infection   166
  microbiology   162-163
  microscopy   164
  persistent conjunctivitis   166-167
  storing and interpreting samples   167
  tests for syphilis   165
  women with possible genital infection 166
contraception   69, 72, 75-81
Data Protection Act 1988   201
detection and management
  commonly sexually transmitted
    organisms   158-159
  genital infections not managed as STIs 158
  incidental findings from urine
    sample/smear   160-161
  knowing which infections are
    sexually transmitted   157-159
  principles   157
  symptomatic patients   159-160
  vertical transmission of infection
    to babies   160
differential diagnosis   160
epidemiological evidence   156
full and appropriate treatment   168
increasing UK rates   155
lack of guidelines for primary care   156
nucleic acid amplification tests   163-164
partner notification   168, 169
patient advice and information   168
referral to GUM   171-174
risk of HIV infection   188
screening for other infections   167
sexual dysfunction   226
supporting quality and audit   176-177
symptoms suggesting   174-176
test of cure   168, 171
transmission prevention   168
useful websites on specific diseases 180-181
vertical transmission to babies   160

SHOW (sexual health outreach worker)
project 29-30
Sieves 236
Sildenafil (Viagra) 216
Smoking
and pregnancy
history-taking 123
cessation advice 127
cessation helplines 135
Specialist young people's services 24
Specificity, of test 236
Spinal injuries, and sexual dysfunction 226
Spermicides *see* Barrier methods
Sterilisation *see* Female sterilisation;
Male sterilisation
Stigma 250
Strand displacement amplification (SDA) 163
Sympto-thermal/multiple index ovulation
method 94
Syphilis (Treponema pallidum) 155
non-treponemal tests 165
partner notification 170, 171
treponemal tests 165

Tadalafil (Cialis) 216
Temperature ovulation method 94
Termination of Pregnancy (Medical Defences)
Act (1995) (Isle of Man) 152-153
Testicular cancer, vasectomy and risk of 101
TFI *see* Tubal factor infertility
Toxic shock syndrome, contraceptive methods
and 77, 93
Travel advice
HIV infected patient 206
COC use and risk of DVT 84
Treponema pallidum (syphilis) 158
sexual transmission 158
see also Syphilis
Triangulation 267
Trichomonas vaginalis infection
COC and reduced risk 77
incidental finding on cervical smear 161
microscopy 164
and preterm birth 160
sexual transmission 159
site of specimen for diagnosis 166
test of cure 171
Tubal clips (rings) 98
Tubal factor infertility (TFI)

prevention
inconsistencies in healthcare delivery 238
see also Chlamydia screening

UKCC for Nursing, Midwifery and Health
Visiting
Code of Professional Conduct and Guidelines
for Professional Practice 140
Under-16s
access to abortion services 141-142
Fraser criteria to assess capacity
to consent 141
see also Young people
Uprima (sublingual apomorphine) 216
Urine samples, STIs detected from 160–161

Vacuum devices 216-217
Vaginal fantasies, sexual dysfunction and 213
Vaginismus 212
Vardenafil (Levitra) 216
Vasectomy 100-101
Venous thromboembolic disease
combined contraceptive patch and 87
COC use and 77, 79, 80, 81, 82, 84
Vestibulitis 212
Viagra (sildenafil) 216
Viral load 189, 190
Vulvodynia 212
Vulvovaginitis 212

Well man/well woman clinics, and chlamydial
screening 238
Wilson and Jungner screening criteria 228, 229
Window period 163, 165, 190

Young people
awareness of general practice
provision 248-249
access to abortion services 140-142
confidentiality of sexual history 42
National Chlamydia Screening
Programme 20, 161
specialist service 24, 28
views about sexual health 248